SYNOPSES IN
UROL

Synopses in Urology

EDITED BY
J.KILIAN MELLON
MD, FRCS(Urol)
Senior Lecturer in Urology,
Department of Surgery,
University of Newcastle upon Tyne
and
Honorary Consultant Urologist,
Sunderland Royal Hospital

ANDREW C.THORPE
MCh, FRCS(Urol)
Consultant Urologist,
Sunderland Royal Hospital

b
**Blackwell
Science**

First published 1998

Set by Setrite Typesetters, Hong Kong
Printed and bound in Great Britain
at MPG Books Ltd, Bodmin, Cornwall

DISTRIBUTORS

Marston Book Services Ltd
PO Box 269
Abingdon, Oxon OX14 4YN
(*Orders*: Tel: 01235 465500
 Fax:01235 465555)

USA
Blackwell Science, Inc.
Commerce Place
350 Main Street
Malden, MA 02148 5018
(*Orders*: Tel: 800 759 6102
 781 388 8250
 Fax: 781 388 8255)

Canada
Login Brothers Book Company
324 Saulteaux Crescent
Winnipeg, Manitoba R3J 3T2
(*Orders*: Tel: 204 224-4068

Australia
Blackwell Science Pty Ltd
54 University Street
Carlton, Victoria 3053
(*Orders*: Tel: 3 9347 0300
 Fax: 3 9347 5001)

The Blackwell Science logo is a
trade mark of Blackwell Science Ltd,
registered at the United Kingdom
Trade Marks Registry

A catalogue record for this title
is available from the British Library
and the Library of Congress

ISBN 0-632-05072-1

Contents

v

List of contributors

I . A P A K A M A , FRCS(Urol)
Consultant Urologist, St George Eliot Hospital, Nuneaton.

N . C H A K O , FRCS(Urol)
Consultant Urologist, Christian Medical Centre, Vellore, India.

S . T . H A S A N, FRCS(Urol)
Consultant Urologist, Sunderland Royal Hospital.

P . M c C A H Y, FRCS(Urol)
Specialist Registrar in Urology, Northern and Yorkshire Region.

J . K . M E L L O N, MD, FRCS(Urol)
Senior Lecturer in Urology, Department of Surgery, University of Newcastle upon Tyne and Honorary Consultant Urologist, Sunderland Royal Hospital.

R . S . P I C K A R D, MD, FRCS(Urol)
Consultant Urologist, Freeman Hospital, Newcastle upon Tyne.

A . S . R O B E R T S O N, FRCS(Urol)
Specialist Registrar in Urology, Northern and Yorkshire Region.

D . J . T H O M A S, MS, FRCS(Urol)
Consultant Urologist, Freeman Hospital, Newcastle upon Tyne and Wansbeck Hospital, Northumberland.

A . C . T H O R P E , MCh, FRCS(Urol)
Consultant Urologist, Sunderland Royal Hospital.

Preface

At present medical education, both at undergraduate and postgraduate level is undergoing major restructuring. For all those training in urology, these changes have heralded an era of more formal assessment of the theory as well as the practice of urology, with new examinations (both compulsory and non-compulsory) with which to contend.

This book is intended to help plug the gap in the present library of urological texts and should be a useful aid to revision in preparation for urological examinations (for both examinees and examiners!). It has a dual function and in addition to being a rapid revision text can provide a framework prior to reading larger standard texts. It is by no means comprehensive and assumes the reader has a basic understanding of core urology. It attempts to cover topics which may be encountered infrequently during training, are currently controversial or are likely to spring to the mind of an examiner.

Many of the references cited in the text (which have been kept to a minimum) are either those papers which are classics from contemporary literature or papers presenting large clinical series, and are hence eminently quotable in the viva situation.

JKM, ACT

Paediatric
Urology

Hypospadias

Definition
- Congenital penile defect, resulting in incomplete development of the anterior urethra.
- Urethra may open anywhere along the ventral shaft of the penis or into the perineum.

Incidence
- Approximately 1 in 300 male births.
- Risk of 6–10% for male siblings and offspring.
- Monozygotic twins, 8.5 times higher risk.

Classifications
Two popular classifications:
1 Browne (1936)
  glanular
  distal penile
  proximal penile
  penoscrotal
  perineal.
2 Duckett (1991)
  anterior (65%)
    glanular (19%)
    coronal (47%)
    distal shaft (34%)
  midpenile (15%)
  posterior (20%).

Clinical features
- Urethral meatus opens over the ventral aspect of the penis or the perineum.
- Abnormal ventral curvature of the penis (chordee).
- Dorsal skin hood (preputial skin).
- Associated anomalies
  cryptorchidism (9.3%)
  inguinal hernia (9.1%)

upper urinary tract anomalies (1–3%).

- Upper urinary tract assessment is particularly indicated in the event of other associated anomalies such as imperforate anus, meningo-myelocele etc.

Management

Corrective surgery may be indicated for cosmetic or functional purposes. The underlying aims are:

- to achieve a straight penis;
- to bring the meatus as close to the normal site as possible;
- to allow a forward directed urinary stream and normal coitus.
  The fundamental surgical steps involve:
- meatoplasty/glanuloplasty
- orthoplasty (penile straightening)
- urethroplasty
- skin cover and scrotoplasty if required.

Surgical treatment

1 Anterior hypospadias
   Meatal Advancement and Glanuloplasty Incorporated (MAGPI):
      particularly for distal defects (complication rate 1–2%).
   Mathieu procedure: for more proximal meatus (complication rate 6%).
   Onlay island flap (using inner preputial skin).
   Glanular Repair and Preputioplasty (GRAP) procedure.
2 Midpenile hypospadias
   Most midpenile defects can be repaired using onlay island flaps (e.g.
      Duckett's island flap).
3 Posterior hypospadias
   Free skin grafts (Devine 1983, preputial skin).
   Vascularized flaps (penile or preputial skin), e.g. Asopa and
      Duckett's transverse preputial island flap, tubular or onlay.
4 Complex hypospadias (hypospadias cripple)
   Bladder mucosal grafts.
   Buccal mucosal grafts.

Further reading

Hendren WH, Reda EF (1986). Bladder mucosa graft for construction of male urethra. *J Ped Surg*, **21**, 189–192.

Duckett JW, Snyder HM III (1992). Meatal advancement and glanuloplasty hypospadias repair after 1000 cases: avoidance of meatal stenosis and regression. *J Urol*, **147**, 665–669.

Gilpin D, Clements WDB, Boston VE (1993). GRAP repair: single-stage reconstruction as an out-patient procedure. *Br J Urol*, 71, 226–229.

Duckett JW, Coplen D, Ewalt D, Baskin LS (1995). Buccal mucosal urethral replacement. *J Urol*, 153, 1660–1663.

British Journal of Urology (1995). Hypospadias. *Br J Urol*, 76 (Suppl. 3).

Epispadias

Definition
- Congenital defect characterized by the urethra opening over the dorsal aspect of the penis in males and by separation of the labia in females.
- Approximately 1 : 117 000 males and 1 : 484 000 females.

Classification
1 Males (depends on site of urethral opening)
  Glanular.
  Penile shaft.
  Penopubic.
2 Females (depends on the degree of the defect)
  Type I: large patulous urethra.
  Type II: near complete split of the dorsal urethra.
  Type III: urethral defect extending proximally involving the sphincter mechanism, usually with exstrophy.

Clinical features
Characteristically in males the dorsal urethral opening is associated with varying degrees of dorsal chordee and a divergent pubic symphysis, whilst in the female the clinical features may include a bifid clitoris, flattening of the mons, separation of the labia and a divergent pubic symphysis.

Commonly associated anomalies
- Deformity of external genitalia.
- Diastasis of the pubic symphysis.
- Deficiency of the continence mechanism.
- Ureteric reflux.
- Rarely, unilateral renal agenesis (usually left).
- Rarely, renal ectopia.

Management

The fundamental aim of reconstructive surgery is to achieve functional and cosmetically acceptable genitalia and effective urinary continence. Various operative techniques are available which can be employed as single or staged procedures. Single stage surgery involves a combined urethral reconstruction (similar to hypospadias repair), a genital reconstruction and bladder neck repair. The Cantwell–Ransley technique is a popular genital reconstruction technique. Briefly, the procedure involves separating the epispadiac penis into individual components and rearranging the dissected components in a more normal anatomical configuration. The Young–Dees and Tanagho are the two bladder neck reconstruction techniques commonly recommended.

Staged repair is usually indicated in complex epispadias particularly associated with exstrophy and a small bladder capacity. The first stage involves urethral and genital reconstruction (as above). Bladder neck repair is performed at a later date to allow bladder growth. Pelvic osteotomy may be required in cases with associated exstrophy. Generally, anterior osteotomy is preferable to posterior.

Most epispadias cases are complex with associated involvement of the sphincter mechanism and exstrophy. Staged repair procedures are therefore preferable.

Further reading

Perovic S, Scepanovic D, Sremcevic D, Vukadinovic V (1992). Epispadias surgery: Belgrade experience. *Br J Urol*, **70**, 674–677.

Gearhart JP, Leonard MP, Burgers JK, Jeffs RD (1992). The Cantwell–Ransley technique for repair of epispadias. *J Urol*, **148**, 851–854.

Gearhart JP, Peppas DS, Jeffs RD (1993). Complete genitourinary reconstruction in female epispadais. *J Urol*, **149**, 1110–1113.

Bladder Exstrophy

Definition

Congenital anomaly presenting with deficient anterior abdominal and bladder walls.

Associated anomalies

- imperforate anus
- inguinal hernia (85%)
- epispadias

- dorsal chordee
- cryptorchidism
- pelvic diastasis
- genital anomalies
  short phallus
  split clitoris
  vaginal and uterine duplication.

The condition can be diagnosed antenatally using ultrasound, which might show little or no bladder filling and an abnormal anterior abdominal wall. Postnatally the diagnosis is clinically obvious.

Management

The aims are to:
- achieve abdominal wall closure;
- provide urinary continence with preservation of renal function;
- construct a cosmetically acceptable phallus in males.

The overall principles of treatment involve adequate counselling for the parents regarding the diagnosis and need for staged repairs which may take years. A staged surgical approach is preferable.
- Ideally the bladder should be closed within the first 24–48 hours of birth, with or without osteotomy (where indicated, anterior innominate is preferable to posterior iliac osteotomy).
- The associated epispadias repair, in males, is usually performed at 2 years.
- Bladder neck repair is performed (Young–Dees–Leadbetter) at 3.5–5 years of age, provided the bladder volume exceeds 60 ml.

Outcome

- Currently the long-term survival rate of children born with bladder exstrophy is >70%.
- Urinary continence can be achieved in over 80% of the cases.
- In patients with exstrophy and incontinent epispadias, primary urinary diversion using Mainz I and Mainz II pouches provides a continence rate of >90% (96% and 97% respectively) with preservation of the upper tracts.
- Although some erectile function is retained in up to 70% of male patients, the majority of patients have retrograde ejaculation.
- Females retain normal fertility.

Association with malignancy

- Bladder exstrophy is associated with a high risk of malignancy.

- Adenocarcinoma is 400 times more common in exstrophy patients.
- Other tumours include squamous cell carcinoma, rhabdomyosarcoma and undifferentiated urothelial carcinoma.

Further reading

Peppas DS, Gearhart JP (1993). Management of bladder exstrophy. In: *Recent Advances in Urology/Andrology*, Vol. 6. (eds WF Hendry, RS Kirby), pp. 63–80. Churchill Livingstone, Edinburgh.

Stein R, Fisch M, Stockle M, Hohenfellner R (1995). Urinary diversion in bladder exstrophy and incontinent epispadias: 25 years of experience. *J Urol*, **154**, 1177–1181.

Cryptorchidism

Introduction

- Incidence: approximately 3–4% of all full-term male births (10% are bilateral).
- Up to 14% have a family history of undescended testis.
- Overall incidence is higher in preterm infants (30%).
- Up to 75% of full-term and 95% of preterm cryptorchids will descend spontaneously by the end of 1 year; most descend by 3 months.
- The incidence, therefore, at 1 year is approximately 0.8%.

Classification

This depends on site of arrest.

- Intra-abdominal: inside the internal inguinal ring.
- Canalicular: between the internal and external inguinal rings.
- Ectopic: away from the normal path of descent.
- Retractile: free moving between the base of the scrotum and the groin.

Investigations

- Herniography: instillation of contrast medium into the peritoneal cavity which enters the hernial sac present in 90–95% of cases. The procedure however is unreliable and invasive.
- Ultrasound: good for canalicular, unreliable for intra-abdominal testis.

- CT scan: better than ultrasound for detection but difficult to perform in infants. In addition, emits radiation.
- MRI: detection rate and difficulties similar to CT but carries significantly less risk for the patient.
- Laparoscopy: currently the investigation of choice. If the intra-abdominal testis is identified orchidopexy can be performed under the same anaesthetic. On laparoscopy, when the processus vaginalis is open approximately 91% of testes are expected to be viable, whereas if it is closed the majority (97%) of testes are either absent or have vanished. In the event of the vas and vessels ending blindly within the abdomen, further exploration is not recommended.

Complications
- Inguinal herniae (patent sac present in 90–95% of cases).
- Testicular torsion may occur, mainly in the postpubertal period; associated with growth of the testis and occasionally with concurrent malignancy.
- Thirty-five to 48 times more likely to develop testicular tumours (seminoma/embryonal cell carcinoma/gonadoblastoma—in intersex). Overall 10% of all testicular tumours arise in cryptorchids; of these, 20% of tumours develop in the contralateral normal testis.
- Other problems include reduced fertility and associated syndromes (Klinefelter's, Noonan's and Prader–Willi's).

Management
Surgical intervention remains the mainstay option in the management of cryptorchidism. Overall aims are to improve aesthetic appearance, place the testis in a palpable location because of risk of associated complications and improve fertility. There is now increasing evidence that early orchidopexy might improve fertility. Ideally the operation should be performed between 12 and 24 months of age. In most cases the testicular pedicle can be mobilized adequately to achieve a one stage orchidopexy. In the event of difficulty with adequate mobilization the Fowler–Stephens principle may be employed, either as a single or staged procedure (division of testicular vessels to improve mobility—testis survives on epididymal and vas deferens blood supply). Recently a further modification has been proposed, the 'Refluo' technique. The technique is based on the observation that testicular loss following the Fowler–Stephens procedure was largely due to venous congestion. The 'Refluo' approach therefore attempts to improve the venous drainage by micro-vascular anastomosis of the testicular vessels to the inferior epigastric

vein and continues to rely on the vasal collaterals for the arterial input. Occasionally when mobilization is not possible autotransplantation may be required, anastomosing the testicular vessels usually to the inferior epigastric vessels.

Other treatment options
- hCG: 3000 IU–40 000 IU, either daily for 7–10 days or weekly for 3 weeks (success rate 14–50% max.).
- LHRH: 1.2 mg/day of a nasal spray for 4 weeks (success rate 6–18% max.).

Further reading
Elder JS (1994). Laparoscopy for impalpable testes: significance of the patent processus vaginalis. *J Urol*, 152, 776–778.
Bianchi A (1995). The impalpable testis. *Ann R Coll Surg Engl*, 77, 3–6.
Docimo SG (1995). The results of surgical therapy for cryptorchidism: a literature review and analysis. *J Urol*, **154**, 1148–1152.
Bukowski TP, Wacksman J, Billmire DA, Lewis AG, Sheldon CA (1995). Testicular autotransplantation: a 17-year review of an effective approach to the management of the intra-abdominal testis. *J Urol*, **154**, 558–561.

Prune Belly Syndrome

Incidence and characteristics
- Almost exclusively in males.
- Approximately 1/35 000–50 000 live births.
- Congenital absence, deficiency or hypoplasia of the abdominal musculature (mainly lower abdominal).
- Large, irregular, thick-walled, hypotonic bladder (with patent urachus).
- Dilated and tortuous ureters (lower ends more severely affected).
- Bilateral cryptorchidism.

Associated anomalies
- Renal dysplasia.
- Hydronephrosis.
- Megalourethra.
- Intestinal malrotation, imperforate anus, gastroschisis, Hirschsprung's disease and occasionally acquired megacolon due to constipation.
- Club foot and compression deformities usually secondary to oligohydramnios.

- Ventricular septal defect, atrial septal defect and tetralogy of Fallot.
- Abnormal seminal vesicles/ducts and prostatic glands.

Management
- Initial neonatal evaluation of cardiopulmonary status is mandatory.
- Evaluate renal function (if stable, observation and surveillance may suffice).
- Deteriorating renal function and/or recurrent urinary tract infection (UTI)—consider cutaneous vesicostomy (Duckett), high loop cutaneous ureterostomy or pyelostomy. In some cases reduction cystoplasty is particularly helpful in the early management of patients with prune belly syndrome by improving voiding and reducing the incidence of urosepsis. In the longer-term, however, it does not seem to normalize voiding dynamics and most patients redevelop large bladder capacities. The procedure should therefore be used with caution in selected cases.
- Additional procedure may include bilateral orchidopexy.
- In most cases abdominal wall defect can be managed using abdominal supports and corsets. In a small number of patients, however, abdominal wall reconstruction (e.g. Monfort's operation) may be necessary.

Further reading
Woodhouse CRJ, Kellett MJ, Williams DI (1979). Minimal surgical interference in the prune belly syndrome. *Br J Urol*, **51**, 475–480.
Parrott TS, Woodard JR (1992). The Monfort operation for abdominal wall reconstruction in the prune belly syndrome. *J Urol*, **148**, 688–690.
Stephens FD, Gupta D (1994). Pathogenesis of the prune belly syndrome. *J Urol*, **152**, 2328–2331.
Bukowski TP, Perlmutter AD (1994). Reduction cystoplasty in the prune belly syndrome: a long-term follow up. *J Urol*, **152**, 2113–2116.

Posterior Urethral Valves

Young's classification
- Type I: obstructing membrane radiating from the inferior aspect of the veru to the membranous urethra.
- Type II: folds radiating cranially from the veru to the posterolateral bladder neck; these are not obstructive.

- Type III: obstructing membrane situated distal to the veru at the level of the membranous urethra.

Clinical presentation
- In severe cases the new born child may present with palpable abdominal masses (bladder, hydronephrosis), ascites, respiratory distress (pulmonary hypoplasia) and associated anomalies, such as Potter's syndrome and positional limb deformities, due to oligohydramnios.
- Milder degrees of obstruction may be detected during early childhood or even at school-going age when children may present with urosepsis, electrolyte abnormalities, failure to thrive and urinary incontinence.

Management
- Prenatal diagnosis is possible using antenatal ultrasound (hydronephrosis, ascites and oligohydramnios).
- Rarely, intervention may be required in the antenatal period using vesico-peritoneal shunts.
- In most cases with significant obstruction a clinical diagnosis is established at birth.
- Providing renal function is stable the infant should be catheterized and antibiotic cover provided.
- Following this, early endoscopic valve destruction can be performed.
- In the event of deteriorating renal function (creatinine >160 µmol/L) a temporary urinary diversion is suggested using cutaneous vesicostomy or ureterostomy (Duckett), followed by endoscopic valve destruction when renal function stabilizes.
- In cases with severe urosepsis, bilateral nephrostomies may be helpful, followed by valve destruction as above when stable.
- In school-going children with mild obstruction and no significant complications, endoscopic valve destruction may suffice.

Outcome
- In the longer-term, approximately 25% of patients with posterior urethral valves develop chronic or end-stage renal failure.
- Overall, patients in whom posterior urethral valves are diagnosed prenatally or shortly after birth are at a higher risk of renal failure compared with those in whom the diagnosis is made later in life.
- It appears that early diagnosis and treatment does not improve prognosis regarding renal failure.

Anterior urethral obstruction

- Congenital urethral obstruction is an uncommon occurrence caused by anterior urethral valves (congenital urethral diverticulum), valvular obstruction of fossa navicularis or cystic dilatation of Cowper's glands (syringocoeles).
- Management of associated urinary obstruction is mainly as described above regarding posterior urethral valves.
- In some cases endoscopic deroofing of the urethral diverticulum and/ or urethroplasty may be required.

Further reading

Parkhouse HF, Barratt TM, Dillon MJ *et al.* (1988). Long-term outcome of boys with posterior urethral valves. *Br J Urol*, **62**, 59–62.

Walker RD, Padron M (1990). The management of posterior urethral valves by initial vesicostomy and delayed valve ablation. *J Urol*, **144**, 1212–1214.

Gonzales ET (1990). Alternatives in the management of posterior urethral valves. *Urol Clin North Am*, **17**, 335–342.

Reinberg Y, De Castano I, Gonzalez R (1992). Prognosis for patients with prenatally diagnosed posterior urethral valves. *J Urol*, **148**, 125–126.

Infection/
Inflammation

Urinary Tract Infections in Childhood

Introduction

- The diagnosis of urinary tract infection (UTI) in the very young is difficult. In infants, non-specific symptoms predominate, e.g. irritability, feeding disorders, vomiting and diarrhoea (occasionally shock, cyanosis or jaundice). Fever, general malaise, frequency, abdominal pain and delayed bladder control are common presenting symptoms in the 1–5 year age group. Children who are 5 years or older have a more typical presentation.
- Symptomatic UTI: 3–5% of girls, 1–2% of boys.
- Age
  < 3 months: M > F;
  3–12 months: M = F;
  > 1 year: F > M.
- Most UTIs are caused by *Escherichia coli*, the remainder by Proteus (especially boys), Klebsiella, Pseudomonas and Enterococcus.
- Commonest underlying cause is urinary stasis due to vesico-ureteric reflux (VUR), detrusor-sphincter dyssynergia, poor bladder emptying habit or constipation. Other causes of stasis include stones, outflow obstruction or secondary to a neurological disorder such as spina bifida.
- It is recommended that all children be investigated after their first confirmed UTI.

UTI, VUR and renal scarring

- Most important outcome of UTI is renal scarring, secondary to renal parenchymal inflammation.
- Scarring (on IVU): 12–20% of children with UTI.
- Scarring (on DMSA scan): 37% of children with UTI.
- The maximal renal inflammatory response to infection is seen at 3–5 days, hence the need for prompt antibiotics.
- 10–20% of children with renal scarring will develop hypertension.
- CPN with renal failure is the commonest reason for renal transplant in children < 19 years in UK.
- VUR
  1–2% of asymptomatic paediatric population;
  30–40% of those with UTI;

90% of those with renal scarring on IVU.
- VUR

  Grade I: reflux into the ureter

  II: reflux into the ureter and pelvis

  III: reflux is associated with mild/moderate dilatation on IVU

  IV: additional blunting of fornices

  V: absent papillary impressions.
- Grades I–III generally resolve spontaneously for about 30–35% of cases each year.
- There may be familial factors for VUR, so some authors recommend investigating siblings.

Risk factors for renal scarring
- severe VUR
- UTI in a child <2 years
- recurrent UTIs
- delayed/inadequate antibiotic therapy.

Management
- Prompt diagnosis. Infant with fever > 38.5°C and no obvious septic focus should have urine cultured and antibiotics commenced. Urine collection can be problematic in very young children. In severely ill children, a catheter sample or suprapubic aspirate may be needed. In a less ill child, a 'clean-catch' or MSU is ideal. If not possible, a bagged sample is recommended (40% false positive rate).
- Prompt treatment with 'best-guess' antibiotic after sending urine for culture. Oral therapy for 5–7 days. Prophylactic antibiotics are then given in low dose at least until investigations are complete.

Radiology
- No single imaging modality provides a complete assessment of the urinary tract.
- USS indicated after a confirmed UTI. However, USS is unreliable in diagnosing VUR or renal scarring, hence other tests are necessary.

Children < 1 year
- Micturating cystogram when urine is sterile to screen for VUR.
- DMSA scan or IVU at 3–6 months following UTI to assess renal damage.

Children >1 year
- Risk of scarring decreases with age and is uncommon after 5 years.
- Micturating cystogram: routine in some centres; in other centres

reserved for systemic infection, previous UTI, recurrent UTI, family history of VUR, abnormal DMSA scan/IVU.
- DMSA scan: routine at 3–6 months after UTI in some centres; other centres are more selective (systemic infection at presentation, previous or recurrent UTI).

Further measures

Improve bladder emptying
- Encourage normal habit.
- Neuropathic bladder: need urodynamics ± intermittent self catheterization.

Long-term, low-dose antibiotics
- Aim to prevent reinfection of the susceptible urinary tract.
- Duration uncertain.
- Usually stopped if all investigations indicate a normal urinary tract.
- With VUR/scarring: continue until 2–3 years old; some centres continue until aged 5–7 years.

Surgery
- Urgent referral if evidence of outflow obstruction or stones.
- VUR: surgery and optimal medical management seem equivalent. Surgery (reimplantation, periureteric injections of teflon or collagen) should be considered if episodes of APN recur despite prophylaxis, on stopping it or if severe reflux is accompanied by a surgically correctable malformation.

Follow-up
- Minimum of 1 year in the very young.
- Usually until the child has been free of infection for 2 years.
- Children with VUR require longer follow-up.
- Annual BP recordings if kidneys scarred.
- Bilateral scarring: annual screening for proteinuria and measurement of renal function for life.
- Advise girls about possible complications during pregnancy (APN, HT, pre-eclampsia).

Further reading
Jacobson SH, Eklof O, Eriksson CG *et al.* (1989). Development of hypertension and uraemia after pyelonephritis in childhood: 27 year follow-up. *Br Med J*, **299**, 703–706.
Smellie JM, Normand ICS, Katz G (1981). Children with urinary infection: a comparison of those with and those without vesico-ureteric reflux. *Kidney Int*, **20**, 717–722.

Smellie JM, Tamminen-Mobius T (1992). Five-year study of medical or surgical treatment in children with severe reflux: radiological renal findings. *Pediatr Nephrol*, **6**, 223–230.

Anonymous (1997). The management of urinary tract infection in children. *DTB*, **35**, 65–69.

Prostatitis

Classification (Drach *et al*. 1978; Table 1)
- Acute and chronic bacterial (ABP and CBP).
- Non-bacterial (NBP)—8 times more common than bacterial.
- Prostatodynia (PD).
- Others: gonococcal, tuberculous, parasitic, mycotic, non-specific granulomatous.

Aetiology
- Similar organisms are seen in bacterial prostatitis as in UTI, e.g. *E. coli*. However, the role of Gram positive bacteria, e.g. *Streptococcus faecalis* is also seen very occasionally in CBP. There are some reports of similar organisms seen in female partners.
- Infection, when present, is probably due to either ascending urethral infection or reflux of infected urine into prostatic ducts. Other possibilities include rectal bacteria from direct spread or lymph invasion
- The cause of NBP and PD is unknown. There may be reflux of urine into prostatic ducts causing a 'chemical' prostatitis.

Diagnosis
- Expressed prostatic secretion (EPS): compare first voided urine and MSU. The EPS normally has <10–20 WBC/hpf. (See Table 1 for findings in various types of prostatitis.) In prostatitis, fat-laden macrophages (oval bodies) are also seen. EPS should never be performed in ABP.
- Bacteriologic localization cultures: ideally these should be performed

Table 1 Common findings in the different types of prostatitis

Type	UTI	Prostate abnormal	WBC in EPS	EPS culture	Organism	Response to antibiotics	Flow rate low
ABP	+	+	+	+	Coliform	+	+
CBP	+	±	+	+	Coliform	+	±
NBP	—	±	+	—	?	—	±
PD	—	—	—	—	?	—	+

at least 5 days post coitus. The bladder should be full and the patient should not have a UTI. The test is performed by collecting and comparing the first voided urine (urethral specimen), MSU, EPS and the last two voids (which represent prostatic samples).

- Immune response: ABP causes an increase in IgG (both serum and prostatic fluid) followed by a slow decrease. Secretory IgA is increased in prostatic fluid for up to 1 year. CBP causes no serum increase in Ig but both IgG and IgA can be increased in the EPS.
- Secretory dysfunction: many changes have been noted in CBP, notably an increased pH. This has important effects on the handling of antibiotics. Decreased prostatic antibacterial activity has also been noted. Further work revealed that this activity was solely due to zinc. The importance of this remains uncertain though treatment with zinc makes no difference.

Acute bacterial prostatitis

The patient presents with fever, chills, low back and perineal pain, dysuria, bladder outflow obstruction and myalgia. Examination reveals pyrexia and on rectal examination the prostate is tender and swollen. Culture of the voided urine should be performed. Urethral instrumentation should be avoided (i.e. retention needs suprapubic catheter).

Pathology

Part or all of the gland is involved with an acute inflammatory reaction. Microabscesses are seen early with large abscesses occurring later.

Treatment

Trimethoprim until C & S available. Appropriate antibiotic for 30 days to prevent CBP.

Chronic bacterial prostatitis

This presents with variable symptoms. There may be irritative voiding with pain in pelvis and/or genitalia. It can present alongside recurrent UTI with the same pathogen (needs localizing techniques). Examination reveals no specific findings, but consider prostatic stones may be involved. These are present in 75% of middle-aged men and 100% of old men. Their cause is either ductal obstruction with hyperplasia or refluxing urine. They cannot be sterilized with medical treatment.

Pathology

Non-specific.

Treatment

Can be either medical or surgical. The former involves long-term antibiotics (4–16 weeks) and has a 30–40% cure rate. If there is no cure then try long-term organism responsive low-dose antibiotics. The surgical option is reserved for highly selected cases but can be useful with stones and involves TURP removing all the infected tissue and stones.

Non-bacterial prostatitis
Presents as for CBP but no bacterial cultures are positive. The cause remains unknown. Some authors feel that *Chlamydia trachomatis* may be involved.

Treatment
This is difficult. A trial of Erythromycin or Tetracycline for 14 days may be helpful. Prostatic massage is of use only for patients with 'congested' prostates who are not undertaking intercourse. There have been reports of success with microwave thermotherapy (see Nickel & Sorensen 1994), otherwise treatment is symptomatic—NSAIDs for pain, anticholinergics for irritative symptoms.

Prostatodynia
This is similar to NBP though men mainly complain of pain which can be in the perineum, groin, testicles, back, suprapubic area, penis and urethra. There is little to find on examination.

Urodynamic investigations show an acquired functional disorder with decreased flow rate and incomplete relaxation of the bladder neck and prostatic urethra. Thus, it may be due to smooth muscle spasm of the bladder neck causing reflux into prostatic ducts and a 'chemical' prostatitis.

Psychological aspects are also thought to be important.

Treatment
As for NBP α-blockers (see Neal & Moon 1994) can be tried, starting at a low dose and then increasing. If beneficial they may be required for life. Psychiatric or psychological help may be required in those who are difficult to treat.

Further reading
Drach GW, Meares EM, Fair WR, Stamey TA (1978). Classification of benign diseases associated with prostatic pain: prostatitis or prostatodynia? *J Urol*, **120**, 266.

Pfau A (1986). Prostatitis. A continuing enigma. *Urol Clin North Am*, **13**, 695–715.

Nickel JC, Sorensen R (1994). Transurethral microwave thermotherapy of non-bacterial prostatitis and prostatodynia: initial experience. *Urology*, **44**, 458–460.

Neal DE, Moon TD (1994). Use of terazosin in prostatodynia and validation of a symptom score questionnaire. *Urology*, **43**, 460–465.

Genitourinary Tuberculosis

Introduction
- Fourteen per cent of non-pulmonary cases of tuberculosis (TB).
- Incidence decreasing (effective treatment of primary TB).
- Overall TB occurrence: 13/100 000 western world; 400/100 000 developing world.
- Genitourinary tuberculosis (GUTB) is caused by dissemination of the organism through the bloodstream and is thus always secondary TB. There is either reinfection or reactivation of old TB.

Pathology

Renal
Blood-borne organisms are deposited close to the glomeruli causing an inflammatory reaction. Macrophages react and granulomas are formed. If bacterial multiplication is checked, fibrous tissue is formed but if it is unchecked, tubercles result with later caseous necrosis. The healing process produces fibrous tissue and then calcium deposition follows. The lesions will eventually slough (*Tuberculous bacilluria*). The disease spreads through the collecting system and once a calyx is stenosed it is rare for the communication to be restored. Calcification is increasing in incidence, though why this should be remains unknown. Hypertension is rarely seen except with extensive renal destruction.

Ureter
This is always an extension of renal TB commonly seen at uretero-vesical junction.

Bladder
Secondary to renal disease. It is seen around the ureteric orifice as inflammation, then bullous granulations and later as ulcers. It then progresses to the muscle which is replaced by fibrous tissue. Tubercles are infrequent.

Testis
Usually secondary to epididymitis.

Epididymis
Blood spread usually to globus minor initially (because of its relatively better blood supply). It can also occur after trauma because of reactivation.

Clinical

- Always consider in patients with vague presentation.
- Thorough family history and past medical history.
- Consider in differential diagnosis when investigating recurrent *E. coli* infection.
- In the developing world, GUTB presents as a more acute illness in young people (male : female = 2 : 1). Superimposed infection is common. It occasionally presents with haemospermia and testicular swelling.

Investigations

- Tuberculin test.
- Urine: ≥3 EMUs.
- Blood: ESR, FBC, U & E.
- XR: KUB (typical appearance of autonephrectomy), CXR, spine.
- IVU: typically shows distorted, lost or deformed calyx/calices. Retrogrades are required for stricture or catheterization.

Management

- Treat active disease. The intentions are to make the patient non-infectious and preserve the maximum amount of renal tissue.
- Short course therapy. Fewer organisms are involved than pulmonary TB and drugs tend to concentrate in urine. For example: Pyrazinamide, Isoniazid, Rifampicin x2/12; then Isoniazid, Rifampicin x2/12.
- Follow-up at 3, 6, 12 months with XRs and EMUs.
- Surgery for GUTB is increasing because although chemotherapy can successfully eradicate bacteria, the complications of the infection remain. Excise diseased tissue, e.g. partial nephrectomy (leaving as much functioning tissue as possible), nephrectomy and epididymectomy. Reconstruct, e.g. ureteric strictures (the role of stents is unknown)—mainly at lower end, augmentation cystoplasty.

Further reading

Anonymous (1991). The management of extrapulmonary tuberculosis. *Drug Ther Bull*, **29**, 26–28.

Gow JG, Barbosa S (1984). Genitourinary tuberculosis. A study of 1117 cases over a period of 34 years. *Br J Urol*, **56**, 449–455.

Schistosomiasis

Introduction

- The bladder disease is due to *Schistosoma haematobium* and was first

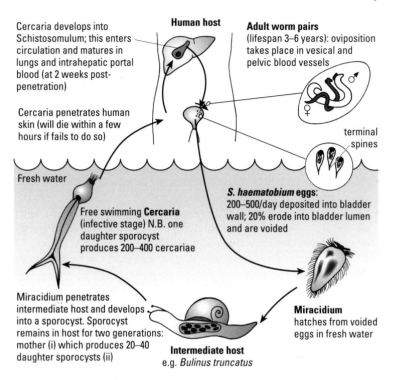

Cercaria develops into Schistosomulum; this enters circulation and matures in lungs and intrahepatic portal blood (at 2 weeks post-penetration)

Human host

Adult worm pairs (lifespan 3–6 years): oviposition takes place in vesical and pelvic blood vessels

Cercaria penetrates human skin (will die within a few hours if fails to do so)

terminal spines

Fresh water

S. haematobium eggs: 200–500/day deposited into bladder wall; 20% erode into bladder lumen and are voided

Free swimming **Cercaria** (infective stage) N.B. one daughter sporocyst produces 200–400 cercariae

Miracidium penetrates intermediate host and develops into a sporocyst. Sporocyst remains in host for two generations: mother (i) which produces 20–40 daughter sporocysts (ii)

Miracidium hatches from voided eggs in fresh water

Intermediate host e.g. *Bulinus truncatus*

Fig. 1 Life cycle of *S. haematobium.*

described by Theodore Bilharz (German pathologist) in Cairo, mid-19th century. Infection with *S. mansoni* and *S. japonicum* mainly involves the colon.
- It is commonly found, and causes significant health problems, in Africa and South-west Asia where an estimated 80–90 million people are infected.
- The life cycle is shown in Fig. 1.
- The adult worms live in the bladder vessels for a mean of 3–4 years but it can be up to 30 years.
- Only 20% of eggs produced by the worms are excreted in the urine, the rest enter the bloodstream or remain within the bladder wall.

Pathology
- Cercarial penetration causes a local immunological reaction (swimmer's itch).
- Disease results from the granulomatous host response to the eggs.
- Syndromes depend on the intensity of infection, the duration, the activity of the disease and the focality.

- The active stage occurs when there are viable adult worms with sustained oviposition and a vigorous granulomatous response (polypoid lesions).
- Disease transmission is possible for up to 13 years.
- The inactive stage occurs when the worms have died and is characterized by 'sandy patches' (calcified eggs in a fibrous matrix).

Clinical
- Swimmer's itch: occurs up to 18 hours after exposure but rarely is the presentation.
- Acute schistosomiasis: a serum-sickness-like illness occurring 3–9 weeks after infection due to active egg laying.
- 'Active' schistosomiasis: presents with terminal haematuria and dysuria. Can persist for years though in a less prominent form when it is known as chronic active schistosomiasis.
- Chronic inactive schistosomiasis: due to complications of the initial disease; obstructive uropathy, recurrent UTIs.

Diagnosis
- Infection: eggs in urine; rectal biopsy (eggs often present in large numbers); ELISA.
- Activity: determined by viability of eggs.
- Intensity: count number of eggs. Egg production has a circadian rhythm with the maximum at noon. Protein excretion parallels that of eggs enabling monitoring with a simple dipstick.

Diagnosis of sequelae
- KUB is the most cost effective method demonstrating calcified bladder and other calcifications.
- IVU is useful for hydroureter etc.
- Cystoscopy should be avoided because of potential complications.

Treatment
- Praziquantel is first line treatment.
- This affects the ion transport mechanism of the schistosome wall causing influx of calcium and sodium with sudden contraction of musculature.
- Eighty to 100% cure.
- Other agents include Metrifonate, Mesylate and Hycanthone.
- Surgery is used for the complications.

Prevention
- No prophylactic drug is currently available. Attempts have been made

to control the disease by targeting aspects of the life cycle, e.g. destroy snails; eliminate contamination of streams/ponds (very difficult); prevent contact with infected water (i.e. better education, particularly of young boys).

Complications
- Bladder cancer: this tends to have an early onset (40–50 years) and is mainly either squamous cell carcinoma or adenocarcinoma (5–15%).
- Urolithiasis: more commonly ureteric then vesical, especially in Egypt.
- Obstructive uropathy: often presents late as it can be silent.
- Bowel problems: polyposis often seen, especially in Egypt. Egg counts increase in the more distal bowel. Heavy infection in appendix can cause appendicitis.
- Potentially many other sites can be involved.

Further reading
El-Sayed HF, Rizkalla NH, Mehanna S, Abaza SM, Winch PJ (1995). Prevalence and epidemiology of *Schistosoma mansoni* and *S. haematobium* infection in two areas of Egypt recently reclaimed from the desert. *Am J Trop Med Hyg*, **52**, 194–198.
Webbe G (1987). Treatment of Schistosomiasis. *Eur J Clin Pharmacol*, **32**, 433–436.
Zaghloul MS (1996). Distant metastasis from Bilharzial bladder cancer. *Cancer*, **77**, 743–749.

Interstitial Cystitis

Introduction
- Interstitial cystitis can only be diagnosed when the typical chronic, irritative voiding symptoms are found with sterile and cytologically normal urine and the characteristic cystoscopic findings (see Gillenwater & Wein 1988).
- It has been known under a number of different names in the past including Hunner's ulcer (1915).
- Female : male ratio is 6–11:1.
- Prevalence of 1–4/10 000.

Aetiology
- Unknown though probably multifactorial.
- Reported increased incidence with HLA-DR6.
- Mast cells have a possible role.
- Deficiency of the normally protective bladder wall glycosaminoglycans.
- Irritants produced in urine.

- Neuropathy (which is probably a secondary process).
- Psychoneurosis.
- There have been extensive attempts to find an infective cause, all of which have failed.

Clinical
- Middle-aged women present with frequency, urgency, nocturia and suprapubic/pelvic pain.
- Physical examination is often normal and no neurological deficit is generally found.

Investigation

Urine
Usually normal. One-third have sterile pyuria. Main differential diagnosis is carcinoma *in situ* so normal cytology should be documented.

Radiology
Not usually required. Investigations should only be performed to exclude other diagnoses.

Urodynamics
Little is gained unless to exclude other diagnoses; record serially to monitor treatment or before undertaking major surgical treatment.

Cystoscopy
Can often look quite normal. Typical finding is 'glomerulation' (pin-point petechial haemorrhage). This can be seen diffusely throughout the bladder on overdistension. These areas should be biopsied. There is often a tinge of blood at end of irrigant emptying and bladders are often of small capacity. The ulcers described by Hunner are seen infrequently.

Histology
The classical appearance was thought to be pancystitis with marked involvement of the deeper layers with inflammation and fibrosis. It is now thought to be inflammation of the urothelium and lamina propria with occasional oedema and mast cells in the muscularis. There is occasional perineural involvement. The changes are generally limited to those cystoscopically abnormal areas. Some authors have demonstrated vasculitis with deposits of Ig and Complement components.

Treatment

- Up to 90% of patients will not require surgery.
- Most authors recommend initial cystoscopy with overdistension which can be repeated (if it works it often only lasts for about 6 weeks or so).
- Intravesical instillation: e.g. dimethyl sulphoxide (DMSO). Can be repeated. Dimethyl sulphoxide has biological actions that include prevention of mast cell degranulation, and it can be added to heparin and steroids.
- Systemic therapy: steroids, calcium channel antagonists, Azathioprine and even Amitriptyline have been shown to have some benefit and should be tried for at least 3 months. Sodium pentosanpolysulphate is currently a popular systemic agent undergoing multicentre clinical evaluation.
- Transcutaneous electrical nerve stimulation (TENS): limited experience to date, though encouraging reports suggest further trials are necessary.
- Surgery: various descriptions of ulcer excision (including laser), denervation procedures, subtotal cystectomy with enterocystoplasty and, as a last resort, urinary diversion and cystectomy. Patient selection is very important and may involve psychological evaluation.

Further reading

Christmas TJ (1991). Interstitial cystitis: immunological aspects and progress in treatment. In: *Recent Advances in Urology/Andrology* 5 (ed. WF Hendry), pp. 103–117. Churchill Livingstone, Edinburgh.

Gillenwater JY, Wein AJ (1988). Summary of the National Institute of Arthritis, Diabetes, Digestive and Kidney Diseases Workshop on Interstitial Cystitis. National Institute of Health, Bethseda, Maryland, August 28–29, 1987. *J Urol*, **140**, 203–206.

Hanno PM (1994). Diagnosis of interstitial cystitis. *Urol Clin North Am*, **21**, 63–66.

Lotenfoe RR, Christie J, Parsons A, Burkett P, Helal M, Lockhart JL (1995). Absence of neuropathic pelvic pain and favourable psychological profile in the surgical selection of patients with disabling interstitial cystitis. *J Urol*, **154**, 2039–2042.

Sexually Transmitted Diseases

Introduction

One sexually transmitted disease (STD) increases the risk of another, including AIDS. Therefore, test and trace contacts. The concepts behind treating STDs successfully are:

- educate the 'at risk' person;
- detect the asymptomatic or non-compliant person;
- ensure effective diagnosis and treatment of the infected individuals;
- evaluate, treat and counsel sexual partners.

The relationship between recurrent STD and subsequent infertility is controversial (see Moskowitz & Mellinger 1992).

Urethritis

Gonococcal urethritis
- The infecting organism is *N. gonorrhoeae.*
- Presents with urethral discharge and burning on micturition.
- Can be asymptomatic in up to 60% of contacts.
- Can improve without treatment but the patient may remain a carrier.
- Prevented by condoms, postcontact antibiotics and intravaginal antiseptics/antibiotics.
- Diagnosis is made from intraurethral swabs (>1 hour postvoid) ± pharyngeal/rectal swabs. They should be plated directly onto Thayer–Martin or New York City media. The organisms will then show on a Gram stain.
- Treatment is with Ciprofloxacillin (single oral dose of 500 mg).

Non-gonococcal urethritis
- Increasing in frequency.
- Fifty per cent or more caused by *C. trachomatis.*
- Thirty to 40% caused by *Ureaplasma urealyticum.*
- In the other cases no cause is found.
- Non-gonococcal urethritis (NGU) is a major cause of cervicitis and the long-term sequelae in women (pelvic inflammatory disease (PID), infertility, ectopic pregnancy and pain) are important.
- Incubation period is 1–5 weeks.
- Diagnosis is by excluding gonococcal urethritis (GU) when patients present with urethritis. When suspected but no inflammation is found, an examination should be performed early in the morning prior to voiding. Culture, if possible, an endourethral swab.
- Treatment is with Tetracycline until cultures are available and then with the appropriate antibiotic. If there is no improvement try Erythromycin. It is important to treat the partner. If problems continue despite the antibiotics, further investigation with flow studies and urethroscopy may be appropriate.

Epididymitis

- Usually caused by spread of infection from urethra or bladder.
- Causes are therefore related to age and sexual orientation: (i) heterosexual <35 years, urethritis common—one-third of acute attacks due to *C. trachomatis*; (ii) homosexual, coliforms commonest; (iii) older men, more commonly associated with bacteriuria secondary to bladder outflow obstruction. (iv) Occasionally epididymitis can be due to systemic diseases, e.g. TB.
- Diagnosis is made by Gram stains of urethral specimens and MSU. White blood cells on urethral smear indicate NGU. The main differential diagnosis in the younger age groups is torsion.
- The treatment is appropriate to the cause.

Genital herpes

- Herpes simplex virus is a double stranded DNA virus.
- Majority due to type I in the UK.
- The first episode is often worse than recurrences and can present with dysuria due to a true urethritis.
- It is possible to isolate the virus.
- Extragenital lesions are possible and rarely neurological complications can occur causing acute retention.
- Diagnosis is made clinically by finding vesicles on an erythematous base.
- Papanicolaou smears show intranuclear inclusions in up to 60% of cases.
- Immunofluorescence reveals 70% of culture-positive cases.
- The only attempt at treatment remains Acyclovir.

Other genital infections

Primary syphilis

- Caused by *Treponema pallidum* (TP).
- The painless 'chancre' appears 2–4 weeks after exposure.
- Diagnosis is made by scrapings or by blood tests: fluorescent treponemal antibody absorption test (FTA-ABS) and microhaemagglutination assay of antibody to TP (MHATP) are fluorescent antibody tests and will remain positive for life; venereal disease research laboratory (VDRL) and the rapid plasma reagin (RPR) tests are non-antibody tests and will therefore correlate with disease activity.
- Treatment is with penicillin (Doxycycline/Erythromycin if sensitive).

Lymphogranuloma venereum
- Caused by *C. trachomatis.*
- Presents with a firm, painless genital papule (occasionally an ulcer) 5–21 days after exposure.
- Often not noticed but usually followed by unilateral inguinal lympha-denopathy and general malaise.
- Diagnosis is by culture from lymph node aspirate.
- Treatment is with Doxycycline.

Chancroid
- Caused by *Haemophilus ducreyi.*
- Presents with a deep genital ulcer.
- Diagnosis is made by Gram stain of material from base of lesion.
- Treatment is with Erythromycin or Cephalosporin.

Granuloma inguinale
- Caused by *Calymatobacterium granulomatis.*
- Initially presents with a small papule that may rarely ulcerate 2–3 months postcontact.
- Later there are subcutaneous granulomatous inguinal swellings that mimic, and can be mistaken for lymphadenopathy.
- Culture of the organism is not possible so diagnosis is made by finding Donovan Bodies (bipolar staining rods) within monocytes.
- Treatment is with Tetracycline or Septrin.

Genital warts
- Caused by human papillomavirus (HPV).
- These have a typical distribution and appearance.
- No cure is possible but local control can be achieved with cryotherapy, podophyllin, diathermy or laser.

Further reading
Moskowitz MO, Mellinger BC (1992). Sexually transmitted diseases and their relation to male infertility. *Urol Clin North Am*, **19**, 35–45.
Taylor-Robinson D (1994). *Chlamydia trachomatis* and sexually transmitted disease. *Br Med J*, **308**, 150–151.

Stone
Disease

Aetiology and Stone Formation

Aetiology

Idiopathic calcium urolithiasis
- Unexplained hypercalciuria.
- Distinguished from primary hyperparathyroidism by normal serum calcium levels.
- Classified as renal (more common in children) or absorptive (adults).
- Approximately 70% of patients with stones belong to this group (renal 10%, absorptive 60%).
- Hyperabsorption of calcium in small intestine inhibits parathormone secretion.
- Renal hypercalciuria results from impaired tubular reabsorption of calcium.
- Metabolic studies reveal a multiplicity of abnormalities, e.g. hypercalciuria, minimal hyperoxaluria, hyperuricosuria, inhibitor deficiency, incomplete renal tubular acidosis.

Hypercalcaemic disorders
1 Primary hyperparathyroidism
    Adenoma or chief cell hyperplasia leads to hypercalcaemia, hypercalciuria and stone formation.
    Hypercalcaemia results from increased synthesis of 1,25-dihydroxycholecalciferol which increases intestinal calcium absorption, renal tubular reabsorption and bone resorption.
2 Prolonged immobilization
    Hypercalcaemia and hypercalciuria result from bone resorption.
3 Milk-alkali syndrome
    Ingestion of large amounts of calcium, vitamin D and alkali may result in hypercalcaemia, alkalosis and possible renal impairment.
    Alkalosis compromises renal excretion of calcium, promoting hypercalcaemic induced soft tissue calcification.
    Nephrocalcinosis and nephrolithiasis may result.
4 Vitamin D intoxication
5 Sarcoidosis
    Non-caseating granulomata produce 1,25 dihydroxycholecalciferol

resulting in increased intestinal calcium absorption and hyper-calcaemia.

6 Disseminated neoplastic disease

7 Cushing's disease

8 Hyperthyroidism

Renal tubular syndromes

1 Renal tubular acidosis

Three types recognized but only type I associated with stone formation.

   Stone formation related to hypercalciuria.

   Relatively alkaline urine.

   Alkaline urine has more divalent/trivalent phosphate ions which combine with calcium, and crystallize.

   Low urinary citrate excretion.

   Mainly pure calcium phosphate stones.

   Nephrocalcinosis occurs.

2 Cystinuria

   Inherited defect of amino acid transport in renal tubules and gastrointestinal tract, involving cystine, ornithine, lysine and arginine (COLA, COAL).

   Autosomal recessive inheritance.

   Three mutated autosomal alleles singly or in combination are responsible for high urinary excretion of these amino acids.

   Relative insolubility of cystine in urine leads to stone formation.

   Family members should be screened with a sodium cyanide-nitroprusside test.

Uric acid lithiasis

- Approximately 5–10% of urinary stones.
- Only develops in humans and Dalmatian dogs.
- Uric acid is an end product of purine metabolism.
- Patients either excrete excessive amounts of uric acid or excessively acid urine.
- Uric acid remains undissociated and insoluble at pH of less than 5.5.
- Hyperuricosuria may be idiopathic or related to enzyme deficiencies which lead to increased *de novo* synthesis of purines that undergo eventual conversion to uric acid.
- Dietary purine and protein excesses may increase urinary uric acid excretion.
- Normal levels of serum and urinary uric acid may be seen in idiopathic uric acid lithiasis.

- Extensive cellular turnover in myeloproliferative diseases or in those receiving chemotherapy may result in increased uric acid production.
- Low urine volumes may be contributory, e.g. in patients with inflammatory bowel disease and ileostomies.

Enzyme disorders

1 Primary hyperoxaluria

Inherited disorder of glyoxalate metabolism (autosomal recessive).

Type I: deficiency of alanine: glyoxalate aminotransferase.

Type II: deficiency of D-glycerate dehydrogenase.

These enzyme deficiencies lead to increased production of endogenous oxalate, the consequences of which are nephrocalcinosis and nephrolithiasis. Patients with primary hyperoxaluria and urinary stone disease often develop evidence of the disease in childhood.

2 Xanthinuria

Rare inherited deficiency of xanthine oxidase.

Stone formation in these patients may be precipitated by allopurinol, a xanthine oxidase inhibitor.

3 2,8-Dihydroadeninuria

An inherited deficiency of adenine phosphoribosyl transferase.

Secondary urolithiasis

1 Secondary hyperoxaluria

Increased enteric oxalate absorption may occur in small bowel resection, inflammatory bowel disease, chronic pancreatitis and jejunoileal bypass.

Either excess fat in the gut binds calcium to form soaps hence reducing the calcium available to bind oxalate and causing increased oxalate absorption, or exposure of colonic mucosa to bile salts with detergent properties increases its permeability to charged ions, including oxalate.

2 Dietary excess

Rhubarb, spinach, kale, tea, cocoa, chocolate, pepper commonly increase urinary oxalate.

3 Infection

Urease producing organisms, e.g. *Proteus*, *Pseudomonas* and *Staphylococcus*, breakdown urea to produce ammonia and CO_2.

Urine becomes alkaline and this promotes formation of struvite calculi (magnesium ammonium phosphate), which may grow to form staghorn calculi.

Escherichia coli never causes struvite stones.

4 Obstruction

 Delayed crystal washout leads to aggregation and stone formation.

5 Medullary sponge kidney

 Twenty per cent of patients with calcium urolithiasis may have this disorder.

6 Urinary diversion

 A combination of infection, acidosis and occasionally stasis.

7 Drugs

 Drugs or their metabolic effects may lead to stone formation, e.g. Acetazolamide stimulates renal tubular acidosis, Allopurinol may precipitate xanthine stones, Thiazide diuretics can result in uric acid stone formation.

Other factors

- geography
- climatic and seasonal factors
- water intake
- diet
- occupation—especially sedentary jobs in hot environment.

Theoretical basis of stone formation

Supersaturation

- This is necessary for stone formation.
- In a supersaturated solution nucleation may occur.
- Nuclei (earliest crystal structure) usually form on existing surfaces such as epithelial lining, cell debris or other crystals (heterogeneous nucleation).
- Occasionally nucleation may occur in free solution (homogenous nucleation).
- Increased number of heterogeneous nuclei may lower the metastable limit of supersaturation (metastable zone = area of supersaturation between the solubility product and spontaneous urinary crystallization for a given substance).
- Microscopic nuclei can aggregate to form large crystalline masses.
- Periods of intermittent supersaturation permit stone formation.
- Epitaxy may promote stone growth (epitaxy is the deposit of one type of crystal on the surface of another type).

Inhibitor deficiency
- Many healthy individuals pass crystals but do not form stones.
- Urine may contain inhibitors of crystal growth and aggregation, e.g. calcium phosphate crystal growth is inhibited by pyrophosphate, citrate and magnesium. Calcium oxalate crystal growth is inhibited by pyrophosphate, citrate and especially glycosaminoglycans.
- Inhibitor deficiency may cause stone formation.
- Kidney proteins inhibit all phases of crystallization.
  Nephrocalcin inhibits calcium oxalate nucleation and aggregation.
  Tamm–Horsfall mucoprotein inhibits aggregation.
  Uropontin inhibits the growth of calcium oxalate crystals.

Crystal retention
- Certain combinations of supersaturation and inhibitor levels permit nucleation and growth of small crystals.
- Most healthy people pass these crystals but some form stones.
- Anatomic abnormalities or adherence to epithelium may prevent these particles from leaving.
- Particle retention may be of free particle (free particles in urine serve as nuclei for further growth of crystals) or fixed particle, e.g. Randall's plaque (due to high concentration in certain areas of the kidney there is precipitation of crystals beneath the surface of papillae).

Matrix
- In addition to crystalline contents calculi contain variable amounts of organic material, i.e. matrix.
- Most solid urinary calculi have a matrix content of about 3%.
- Matrix calculi composed of an average of 65% of matrix by weight may occur, especially in association with urinary infection.
- Chemical analysis of matrix reveals it to be 65% hexosamine and 10% bound water.
- Whether matrix truly initiates stone formation or plays a part in causation of stone disease remains uncertain.

Further reading
Anonymous (1990). Update on urinary stone disease. *Urol Clin North Am*, 17, 157–242.

Coe FL, Parks JH, Asplin JR (1992). The pathogenesis and treatment of kidney stones. *N Engl J Med*, 327, 1141–1152.

Cohen TD, Ehreth J, King LR, Preminger GM (1996). Pediatric urolithiasis: medical and surgical management. *Urology*, 47, 292–303.

ESWL in Treatment of Urinary Calculi

Introduction
- Non-invasive method of treatment by generating shock waves outside the body which are focused on stones.
- First successful treatment was in February 1980 at the University of Munich using the Dornier Human Model-1 (HM-1).

Mechanism of action
- A high energy amplitude of pressure (shock wave) is generated by an abrupt release of energy in a small space.
- Waves are transmitted with little attenuation through water and soft tissues.
- When the wave encounters a boundary between substances of different densities or acoustic impedance, e.g. a stone, the pressure front is partially reflected at the front surface and splits into compressive and tensile components. A high pressure gradient develops owing to these two forces and disintegration begins on the stone surface closest to the shock wave source. Part of the wave continues through the stone and on reflection from the distant surface similar forces develop. The compressive/tensile phenomenon results in an implosion rather than explosion, hence the low incidence of adjacent tissue injury. Disintegration of outer layers exposes the inner layers which in turn are broken up. Cavitation also occurs and helps stone disintegration.

Generation

Spark gap
Generated under water by an electric spark gap of 15–25kV. The high voltage spark is discharged under water and causes rapid evaporation of water which generates a shock wave by expanding the surrounding fluid. The generator is located at one focal point of an ellipsoid (F1) which focuses the shock wave to a second focal point (F2). Coupling is by a water cushion. Shock waves generated in this fashion must be co-ordinated with an ECG monitor to prevent cardiac arrhythmias.
Examples: Dornier HM-3, Medstone STS, Technomed Sonolith.

Electromagnetic
Electric currents move a metal membrane within a rigid shock tube to generate shock waves. Focused by an acoustic lens to F1 at the stone site. Coupling is by a water cushion.

Examples: Siemens Lithostar, Storz Modulith.

Piezoelectric
Piezoceramic elements are placed on a concave reflector. These are excited by a high frequency, high voltage energy pulse. Motion of the elements generates an ultrasonic wave which is focused to F1. Wide aperture and a small focal point results in anaesthesia free use.
Examples: EDAP LT-01, Wolf Piezolith.

Microexplosive
Generated by controlled microexplosion using lead azide pellets and focused by an ellipsoid. Coupling is by a water bath.
Example: Yachiyoda SZ-1.

Stone localization
- plain X-ray (Medstone STS)
- fluoroscopy
- ultrasound.

Bioeffects
- Haematuria (nearly universal following ESWL).
- Perirenal haematoma/oedema.
- Parenchymal haemorrhage (probable explanation of haematuria).
- Parenchymal oedema.
- Tubular necrosis possibly causing subsequent fibrosis.
- Permanent decrease in renal function is uncertain.
- Hypertension is uncertain.

Special considerations
- Stents: do they encourage or impede passage of fragments? May help localization and create a fluid interface around ureteric stones.
- Pacemakers: is ESWL safe with cardiac pacemakers? Damage to pacemakers could occur by electromagnetic interference or mechanically. Pretreatment assessment by cardiologist, or cardiologist in attendance during treatment may be necessary. May need to deprogramme pacemaker during treatment.

Further reading
Anonymous (1990). Update on urinary stone disease. *Urol Clin North Am*, **17**, 157–242.

Drach GW, Weber C, Donovan JM (1990). Treatment of pacemaker patients with extracorporeal shock wave lithotripsy: experience from two continents. *J Urol*, **143**, 895–896.

Schulze H, Hertle L, Kutta A, Gratt J, Senge T (1989). Critical evaluation of treatment of staghorn calculi by percutaneous nephrolithotomy and extracorporeal shock wave lithotripsy. *J Urol*, **141**, 822–825.

Lingeman JE, Woods JR, Toth PD (1990). Blood pressure changes following extracorporeal shock wave lithotripsy and other forms of treatment for nephrolithiasis. *JAMA*, **263**, 1789–1794.

Nakada SY, Pearle MS, Soble JJ, Gardner SM, McClennan BL, Clayman RV (1995). Extracorporeal shock wave lithotripsy of middle ureteral stones: are ureteral stents necessary? *Urology*, **46**, 649–652.

Ureteronephroscopy for Stone Disease

Introduction

- Advances in design of endoscopes for ureteronephroscopy have rendered the entire urinary tract accessible to endoscopic examination and manipulation.

History

- First endoscopy of the ureter was by Hugh Hampton Young (1912) who passed a paediatric cystoscope into a dilated ureter and renal pelvis of a child with posterior urethral valves.
- Became an accepted technique after independent reports by Goodman (1977) and Lyon and coworkers (1978).

Instruments

- Rigid: various makes and sizes; the instrument channels vary in size and in number and in whether the channel is straight or curved. Ultrasound probes require straight channels but the lithoclast will pass through a gentle curvature.
- Semirigid: e.g. Candela miniscope—7.2F, 43 cm long, 2 channels (2.0/3.2F).
- Flexible: the only true ureteronephroscope. Can be actively deflectable or passive. Former is more expensive but with passive instrumentation there is no means of manoeuvring on to a stone. Poorer resolution, smaller working channels.

Ureteric dilatation

- Wire guided: placement more accurate with certainty of entering and remaining within lumen as guide wire is passed first. Followed by use of olive tipped metal bougies, graduated flexible dilators or balloon dilatation.

- Non-guided: successively larger semirigid catheters or bougies are passed under endoscopic control.

Treatment of calculi
- Direct retrieval for calculi < 6 mm using basket, snare or wire graspers.
- Ultrasonic lithotripsy: ultrasound generator produces ultrasound waves which are transmitted down a hollow or solid probe. The vibrating action at the tip of the probe in contact with the stone produces a drilling or grinding action which results in stone pulverization. Used with rigid scopes. Can cause thermal damage to the ureter.
- Electrohydraulic lithotripsy (EHL): electrically generated spark at the tip of the probe causes momentary heat in a localized area. Small amount of irrigant is vaporized forming a gas bubble. The bubble, as it expands, creates a hydraulic shock wave that impacts on the stone. The entire sequence occurs in $1/800^{th}$s. Probe placed on, or not more than 1 mm from stone. Risk of ureteric perforation is a disadvantage.
- Laser lithotripsy: Nd:YAG, holmium, pulsed-dye or Alexandrite laser. When probe is discharged in direct contact with stone, a plasma (ionized gas) develops on the surface of the stone. As the laser is repeatedly fired the plasma absorbs more laser energy and rapidly expands, thereby creating a shock wave that audibly impacts on the stone.
- Lithoclast: uses compressed air to activate a solid probe in a manner similar to a jackhammer. Good stone fragmentation but rigid probe design limits use to rigid endoscopes. Safe modality but imparts greatest propulsion to the stone.
- Electrokinetic lithotripsy (EKL).

Success rates
- overall 70–80%
- rigid
  lower ureter 93–99%
  midureter 66–83%
  upper ureter 33–78%
- flexi
  70–85%.

Complications
- perforation
- extravasation
- mucosal damage
- avulsion
- haematuria
- infection
- stricture
- instrument breakage.

Further reading

Coptcoat MJ, Ison KT, Watson G, Wickham JE (1988). Lasertripsy for ureteric stone in 120 cases: lessons learned. *Br J Urol*, **61**, 487–489.

Denstedt JD, Clayman RV (1990). Electrohydraulic lithotripsy of renal and ureteral calculi. *J Urol*, **143**, 13–17.

O'Keefe NK, Mortimer AJ, Sambrook PA, Rao PN (1993). Severe sepsis following percutaneous or endoscopic procedures for urinary tract stones. *Br J Urol*, **72**, 277–283.

Dretler SP (1994). Ureteroscopic fragmentation followed by extracorporeal shock wave lithotripsy: a treatment alternative for selected large or staghorn calculi. *J Urol*, **151**, 842–846.

Percutaneous Stone Surgery

Introduction
- First performed in 1976 by Fernstrom and Johannson who were the first to use an elective percutaneous nephrostomy tract to enter a calculus-containing kidney and remove the stone.
- Wickham and Kellet in 1981 reported the first 31 cases of totally elective nephrolithotomy and the method was given the name percutaneous nephrolithotomy (PCN, or more recently PCNL).

Indications
- Obstruction: anatomic abnormalities such as PUJ obstruction, calyceal diverticula or ureteric obstruction may prevent stone fragments passing post-ESWL.
- Stone bulk > 3 cm or staghorn.
- Anatomic abnormalities such as large patient bulk when stone cannot be placed in the focal point of ESWL machine.
- Stone location: lower calyceal stones are less likely to pass, especially in a dilated system.

- Stone composition: struvite stones need to be completely removed because of infection. Also, some stones are difficult to pulverize using ESWL but may be broken sufficiently by PCNL for fragments to be removed, e.g. calcium oxalate monohydrate, cystine stones.

Complications
- injury to spleen, pleura, colon
- haemorrhage
- sepsis
- extravasation
- retained fragments
- difficult subsequent open surgery.

Special circumstances
- Complex and staghorn calculi: Y-puncture may be required.
- Calyceal diverticula: the puncture must be on to the diverticulum.
- Horseshoe kidney: due to malrotation a more medial tract is used. Longer Amplatz sheaths and longer endoscopes.
- Transplants: where ureter is difficult to catheterize ultrasound guided puncture is an option.
- Children: difficulty with ureteric catheterization may dictate either ultrasound guided puncture or fluoroscopy puncture with IVU guidance.
- Ureteric stones: a higher placed puncture may be needed to permit antegrade ureteroscopy.

Staghorn calculi
- Complete endoscopic stone removal if possible.
- PCNL for debulking followed by ESWL. The advantage of this is the reduced need for additional renal access and secondary endourologic procedures.

Further reading
O'Keefe NK, Mortimer AJ, Sambrook PA, Rao PN (1993). Severe sepsis following percutaneous or endoscopic procedures for urinary tract stones. *Br J Urol*, **72**, 277–283.

Lingeman JE, Siegel YI, Steele B, Nyhuis AW, Woods JR (1994). Management of lower pole nephrolithiasis: a critical analysis. *J Urol*, **151**, 663–667.

Lam HS, Lingeman JE, Mosbraugh PG *et al.* (1992). Evolution of the technique of combination therapy for staghorn calculi: a decreasing role for extracorporeal shock wave lithotripsy. *J Urol*, **148**, 1058–1062.

Medical Management

Introduction
- Goal is mainly to prevent formation of new stones or the further growth of existing stones.
- It has to be effective and continuous and may require lifelong treatment.
- High fluid intake is generally advised.
- Prevent supersaturation.
- Aim is to produce at least 2500 ml of urine in 24 hours.
- Dietary history is taken and excesses are eliminated.

Idiopathic calcium lithiasis
- Increased fluid intake and correction of dietary excesses (of calcium and oxalate).
- Thiazide diuretics may reduce urinary calcium excretion by increasing fractional calcium reabsorption in the distal nephron.
- Orthophosphates may be used, which decrease urinary calcium excretion and increase inhibitor activity.
- Cellulose phosphate given enterally is useful in absorptive hypercalciuria. It is a calcium binding resin and reduces calcium absorption when taken with meals.
- Citrate mixtures are used to increase inhibitor activity in urine.

Hypercalcaemic disorders
- Increased fluid intake may prevent calculus formation, especially in immobilized patients.
- Oral orthophosphates may be used to decrease urinary calcium excretion.
- Corticosteroids in sarcoidosis reduce serum calcium.
- Thiazide diuretics.

Renal tubular acidosis
- Sodium or potassium bicarbonate or citrate is given resulting in an increased renal citrate excretion.

Cystinuria
- Citrate preferred to bicarbonate.
- Aim is to increase urinary pH to 7.5–7.8.
- D-penicillamine may be used. Reacts with cysteine to form a soluble salt that reduces, through competition, the formation of cystine. It is

a potentially toxic drug and should only be used if hydration and alkalinization fail. Adverse effects include rashes, fever, agranulocytosis, arthralgia and lymphadenopathy.

- α-mercaptopropionylglycine (MPG) is an alternative and has fewer side effects.
- Captopril may also be used. May lower urinary cystine levels in homozygous cystinuric patients. Mechanism unknown. Can cause orthostatic hypotension.
- Dietary methionine (precursor of cystine) restriction rarely needed.

Uric acid lithiasis
- Uric acid stones may be dissolved medically.
- Urinary pH is increased to 6.5 using bicarbonate or citrate.
- Allopurinol, a xanthine oxidase inhibitor, may reduce uric acid excretion; once calcium is dissolved this is discontinued and alkalinization maintained.

Primary hyperoxaluria
- Large doses of pyridoxine reduce urinary oxalate excretion in 20–50% of patients.
- Neutral orthophosphates may be used to halt the growth of existing calculi.

Enteric hyperoxaluria
- Fat restriction is necessary.
- Oral calcium supplements indicated.
- Cholestyramine may be used to bind acidic components in the gut lumen including oxalate.
- Intestinal bypass may need to be reversed.

Stones associated with infection
- After surgical removal, antimicrobial prophylaxis should be maintained for 3–12 months.
- Urinary acidification with ammonium chloride may be used in conjunction.
- Dissolution of stones with Hemiacidrin or Suby G and M solutions is an option.

Further reading
Yu TF (1981). Urolithiasis in hyperuricaemia and gout. *J Urol*, **126**, 424–430.
Smith LH (1989). The medical aspects of urolithiasis: an overview. *J Urol*, **141**, 707–710.

Seftel A, Resnick MI (1990). Metabolic evaluation of urolithiasis. *Urol Clin North Am*, **17**, 159–169.

Cicerello E, Merlo F, Gambaro G *et al.* (1994). Effect of alkaline citrate therapy on clearance of residual renal stone fragments after extracorporeal shock wave lithotripsy in sterile calcium and infection nephrolithiasis patients. *J Urol*, **151**, 5–9.

Coe FL, Parks JH, Asplin JR (1992). The pathogenesis and treatment of kidney stones. *N Engl J Med*, **327**, 1141–1152.

Cohen TD, Ehreth J, King LR, Preminger GM (1996). Pediatric urolithiasis: medical and surgical management. *Urology*, **47**, 292–303.

Trauma and Reconstruction

Complications Following Urinary Intestinal Diversion

Metabolic
Electrolyte abnormalities depend upon the bowel segment utilized
* Stomach: hypochloraemic metabolic alkalosis.
* Jejunum: hyponatraemic, hyperkalaemic metabolic acidosis.
* Ileum and colon: hyperchloraemic metabolic acidosis (may also get hypokalaemia, hypomagnesaemia, hypocalcaemia, hyperammonaemia, raised creatinine and urea).

Jejunum
Abnormalities result from:
* increased secretion of sodium and chloride which also carries water with it;
* increased rennin and aldosterone.
The patient may become grossly dehydrated and hypovolaemic.

Ileum and colon
Acidosis develops to some degree in most patients, but is usually minor in 60–70%. Severe acidosis and electrolyte disturbances are rarer; 10–18% in small bowel cystoplasties but up to 80% in ureterosigmoidostomies.
* In continent diversion involving ileum and caecum or caecum alone, the majority of patients get raised sodium chloride and depressed bicarbonate.
* Mainz pouch: 65% require alkali therapy to maintain normal acid–base balance.
* If small bowel alone is used there are electrolyte disturbances in 10–15% of cases.
* Treatment of hyperchloreamic metabolic acidosis involves either alkalizing and/or chloride transport blockers.
* Oral sodium bicarbonate is effective but not well tolerated—produces excess intestinal gas. Alternatives include sodium citrate, citric acid or polycitra (includes potassium citrate as well).
* Patients with persistent acidosis, in whom large sodium loads are undesirable may need Chlorpromazine or nicotinic acid (chloride transport blockers). These limit acidosis but will not fully correct it.

- Hypokalaemia and total body depletion of potassium may occur in urinary intestinal diversion; this is commonest in ureterosigmoidostomies. Body potassium may be reduced by 30%—probably due to renal wasting of potassium secondary to renal damage. The ileum is more likely to reabsorb potassium when present in higher concentration in the urine than colon, hence the reason why more problems occur with potassium in ureterosigmoidostomies and ureterocolonic diversions.
- Urea and creatinine are both reabsorbed by ileum and colon, so their serum concentrations are not a true reflection of renal function.

Histological alteration of intestine secondary to chronic urine exposure

- Villous atrophy and pseudocrypt formation, especially in the ileum. These changes are patchy, not affecting all of the bowel in the diversion.
- Submucosal inflammatory infiltrates. In general there are fewer changes in colonic mucosa over the long term, but there is a decrease in goblet cell size. Changes occur in active transport systems in the brush border.

Altered sensorium

- This is due to alteration in ammonia metabolism, leading to ammoniagenic coma in patients with cirrhosis, altered liver function and in some patients with normal liver function.
- This is most commonly seen after ureterosigmoidostomies and is treated by conduit drainage or diversion drainage, oral neomycin to decrease enteric load and decrease protein consumption and, in severe cases, arginine gluconate with 11 5% dextrose.

Abnormal drug absorption

Problems occur with drugs absorbed by the gastrointestinal (GI) tract and then excreted unmetabolized by the kidney.
These include:

- phenytoin
- several antibiotics
- methotrexate in patients with ileal conduits
- patients with continent diversion receiving chemotherapy should be put on to constant drainage.

Osteomalacia

This has been reported in patients with cystoplasties, ileal conduits, colonic conduits and ileal ureters, but is most common in ureterosigmoidostomies.

- Acidosis causes excess protons to be buffered by bone with calcium release.
- Correcting the acidosis does not always remineralize bone.
- Some patients exhibit vitamin D resistance which is independent of the acidosis; this is probably renal in origin and is usually overcome by using 1-α-hydroxycholecalciferol.
- Increased sulphate reabsorption from conduit pouches inhibits calcium and magnesium reabsorption and results in their loss from the kidney.

Growth and development

- Urinary diversion is detrimental to growth and development causing a decrease in linear growth.
- Many patients with diversion fall far below the 10th centile for growth compared to control patients on intermittent self catheterization only, with no surgery.

Infection

There is increased evidence of bacteriuria, bacteraemia and sepsis in patients with bowel interposition.

- A significant number of patients with intestinal cystoplasties develop pyelonephritis.
- Acute pyelonephritis is reported in 10–17% of patients with colonic or ileal conduits.
- Four per cent of patients with ileal conduits die from sepsis (Schmidt *et al.*).
- Seventy-five per cent of ileal conduit samples are infected, but most cases are asymptomatic.
- Deterioration in upper tracts is more commonly associated with *Proteus* or *Pseudomonas*.
- Sixty-six per cent of patients with Kock's continent pouches have positive cultures—the small intestine is probably unable to inhibit bacterial proliferation, unlike urothelium. Intestine makes urine less bacteriostatic and may promote bacterial growth.

Short bowel and nutritional problems

- Significant terminal ileum loss leads to vitamin B_{12} malabsorption.
- If bile salts enter the colon due to ileal surgery this will lead to

irritation of colonic mucosa and diarrhoea; the 'Ileal break' mechanism may be lost.

- Normally when lipid comes into contact with ileal mucosa, motility decreases so that absorption will increase. However, as a result of ileal resection unmetabolized lipids reach the colon resulting in diarrhoea.

Loss of the ileocaecal valve

- There is bacterial reflux into the ileum interfering with fatty acid reabsorption and bile salt interaction.
- Vitamin B_{12} absorption is also affected.
- Lack of fat absorption also decreases absorption of other fat soluble vitamins—A and D.

Loss of jejunum
Affects:

- fat metabolism
- calcium metabolism and folic acid.

Loss of colon

- Diarrhoea due to lack of fluid and electrolyte absorption.
- Bicarbonate loss due to increased secretion in ileum.

Miscellaneous

Incidence of stones

- Colonic conduits 3%.
- Ileal conduits 10–12%.
- Continent caecal reservoir 20%.

These are mainly triple phosphate, but calcium oxalate stones occur in short bowel syndrome.

Uretero–small bowel anastomosis

- Bricker, described 1950.
- Wallace, described 1970, has the lowest of all complications (stricture 3%, upper tract dilatation 4%, leakage 2%).

Cancer in ureterosigmoidostomies

- Incidence 6–29%, mean 11% (Zabbo & Kay 1986).
- Occurs at 5–50 years, mean 21 years.
- Types: adenocarcinoma, transitional cell carcinoma and sarcoma (nitrosamines are the probable promoter of cancer).

Further reading

Golimbu M, Morales P (1975). Jejunal conduits: technique and complications. *J Urol*, **113**, 787–795.

Schmidt JD, Hawtrey CE, Flocks RH *et al.* (1973). Complications, results and problems of ileal conduit diversions. *J Urol*, **109**, 210–216.

Ashken MH (1987). Urinary caecal reservoir. In: *Bladder Reconstruction and Continent Urinary Diversion.* (eds LR King, AR Stone, GD Webster), pp. 238–251. Year Book Medical Publishers, Chicago.

Bricker EM (1950). Bladder substitution after pelvic evisceration. *Surg Clin North Am*, **30**, 1511–1521.

Zabbo A, Kay R (1986). Ureterosigmoidostomy and bladder exstrophy. A long term follow up. *J Urol*, **136**, 396–398.

Cohen MS, Hilz ME, Davis CP *et al.* (1987). Urinary carcinogens (nitrosamine) production in a rat model for ureterosigmoidostomy. *J Urol*, **138**, 449–452.

Nurse DE, Munday AR (1989). Metabolic complications of cystoplasty. *Br J Urol*, **63**, 165–170.

Management of the Ruptured Bladder

Bladder rupture is associated with other injuries in 85% of cases when it is secondary to external trauma, hence the high mortality rate of 22–44%. The treatment of associated injuries takes precedence over the bladder.

Early symptoms and signs
- Bruising over lower abdomen, guarding and rigidity.
- With bladder contusions patients are able to void but may have macro- or microscopic haematuria.
- With ruptured bladder patients are unable to void.
- In multiple injuries with blood at the external meatus an ascending urethrogram is mandatory to rule out associated urethral trauma.

Late symptoms and signs
- acute abdomen
- absence of voiding
- increased urea in serum

Late presentation is usually associated with increased alcohol consumption and domestic violence.

Radiological evaluation
- If urethral trauma is suspected an ascending urethrogram is performed first followed by a retrograde cystogram washout film.

- Bladder rupture is associated with posterior urethral injuries in 10–29% of cases.
- In all patients with a pelvic fracture and posterior urethral rupture the index of suspicion of bladder rupture should be high.
- In extraperitoneal bladder rupture there is no increase in serum urea.
- With intraperitoneal bladder rupture the urea rises rapidly (within 30 minutes in simulated bladder rupture in animals).

Association with pelvic fractures
Pelvic fractures are associated with 83% of ruptured bladders.
- Fractured pubic rami (55%).
- Fractured anterior and posterior pelvic ring (12%).
- Comminuted fractures (12%).
- Acetabular fractures (11%).

Flaherty has reported a significant correlation between injury to the bladder and posterior urethra, and the extent of pelvic ring disruption.
- There is an incidence of 8% lower urinary tract injury in all pelvic fractures.
- The bladder may be damaged iatrogenically during manipulation of a pelvic fracture.

Retrograde cystography
- A simple contusion will show compression or lateral displacement of the bladder.
- For both extra- and intravesical rupture, cystogram technique is vitally important. At least 400 ml of contrast under gravity fill are infused, the bladder is then emptied and a washout film performed. If less than 400 ml is used a significant false negative rate will occur, because sharply cut edges, elasticity of the bladder wall, oedema and interlacing detrusor fibres will cause coaptation and prevent any extravasation.

Extraperitoneal bladder rupture
Shearing forces produced during a pelvic fracture will tear the bladder at its moorings (laterally and basally to the bony pelvis). This usually causes an extraperitoneal (EP) rupture.
- In a report of 200 pelvic fractures and 100 bladder ruptures, EP bladder rupture was seen without pelvic fracture in only three cases (Corriere); all ruptures were due to blunt trauma.

Investigations
An ascending urethrogram and static cystogram should be performed.
- 'Flame shaped' contrast denotes an EP rupture.
- If a complex EP rupture has occurred, extravasation beyond the confines of the pelvis, e.g. scrotum, penis, thigh etc., may occur.
- A large haematoma will cause a 'tear-drop' bladder.

Treatment
- The volume of extravasation does not correlate with size of rupture.
- Corriere studied 41 patients treated by catheter drainage (32 penile, 9 suprapubic) for at least 10 days; all healed, including those with complex extravasation.
- If the patient is undergoing a laparotomy for concomitant trauma, do not disturb any pelvic haematoma but open the bladder dome and repair any tear intravesically. Leave in a suprapubic catheter.
- The mortality rate is 12% from associated injuries (visceral and vascular).
- Perform a cystogram before removal of the suprapubic catheter.

Complications
These are usually related to delay in diagnosis and include sepsis, uroascites and peritonitis if intraperitoneal (IP) rupture is also present.

Intraperitoneal bladder rupture
The pressure required to rupture a normal healthy bladder exceeds 300 cm H_2O. IP rupture occurs secondary to:
- decelerating injury (road traffic accidents)
- penetrating (knife) injuries
- pelvic fractures secondary to a fall.

Table 2 Site of rupture in 293 patients

	EP	IP	Both
Corriere and Sandler	62	34	9
Cass	76	53	8
Carrol and McAninch	32	13	6
Total	170(58%)	100(34%)	23(8%)

Diagnosis

A careful history and examination, retrograde urethrogram and cystogram with adequate bladder distension will be required.

- Missed diagnosis may lead to uraemia and a mild acidosis.

Treatment

Exploration, repair of rupture and suprapubic drainage are mandatory.

- Twenty per cent of mortality is due to associated visceral and vascular injuries.
- Evaluation of the upper as well as lower urinary tract is essential before exploration.
- Follow-up cystogram at 2 weeks postop. If no extravasation is seen the suprapubic catheter should be clamped and if the patient voids the catheter removed.
- Persistent suprapubic drainage with residual urine suggests voiding dysfunction or outflow obstruction.

Complications

- Persistent suprapubic drainage.
- Pelvic abscess between rectum and prostate.
- In patients presenting with a ruptured bladder and a raised white cell count over 20 000, the additional injury of a ruptured spleen should be suspected.

Further reading

Cass AS (1989). Diagnostic studies in bladder rupture: indications and techniques. *Urol Clin North Am*, 16, 267–273.

Palmer JK, Benson GS, Corriere JN (1983). Diagnosis and initial management of urological injuries associated with 200 consecutive pelvic fractures. *J Urol*, 130, 712–14.

Corriere JN, Sandler CM (1989). Management of extraperitoneal bladder rupture. *Urol Clin North Am*, 16, 275–277.

Peters PC (1989). Intraperitoneal rupture of the bladder. *Urol Clin North Am*, 16, 279–282.

Acute Urethral Injuries and Posterior Urethral Stricture Repair

Introduction

A clinical diagnosis of urethral rupture is made on finding blood at the urethral meatus, a palpable bladder and an inability to void. Secondary features are a high riding prostate on rectal examination and perineal haematoma. There is no place for diagnostic catheterization—this may turn a partial tear into a full rupture, increase haemorrhage from the prostatic bed and infect a previously sterile haematoma. Absence of signs does not preclude a urethral injury.

Urethrography
- Insert a 16 or 18 Foley catheter with 1–2 ml in the balloon into the fossa navicularis.
- Place the patient at 25–35°, inject 20–25 ml of contrast and use fluoroscopy.
- Do not use the antero-posterior view; this foreshortens the bulbar urethra which superimposes upon itself masking extravasation.
- If a catheter has already been passed do not remove it as this has virtually excluded a complete rupture and any small tears will heal; perform voiding urethrography on removal of the catheter.

Classification of urethral injuries

Anterior
Penile and bulbar: associated with straddle injuries.

Posterior
Membranous and prostatic: associated with pelvic fractures.
- Posterior injuries occur in 5% of males with pelvic fractures.
- Classically the prostatomembranous urethra is ruptured above the urogenital (UG) diaphragm; extension of the injury into the bulbar urethra or rupture of the UG diaphragm is rare.
- When the prostate is sheared from its connection to the UG diaphragm, urinary extravasation will not occur, unless the bladder neck has been previously compromised and disrupted.
- Urethrography will show extravasation in the prostatic bed and the perivesical space. It is limited inferiorly by the UG diaphragm.
  Three subgroups of posterior urethral injury are described (Colapinto & McCallum).
- Type I: no rupture of urethra. The puboprostatic ligaments are ruptured. Haematoma occurs in the prostatic fossa and the bladder base becomes elevated leading to a stretched posterior urethra.
- Type II: urethral disruption occurs at the prostatomembranous junction above UG diaphragm. Contrast is extravasated into the extraperitoneal space above an intact UG diaphragm. This is the classical injury.

- Type III: disruption of the membranous urethra with extension of injury into the proximal bulb. Contrast extravasates below the UG diaphragm into the perineum.

Despite the classical description 60 to 90% of patients have a type III injury on urethrography, according to Colapinto. Webster reviewed 274 patients (nine series) and found that 34% of ruptures were partial—these are important injuries and most will result in short strictures which will be amenable to non-open operative therapy. Complete rupture usually results in a long stricture requiring open surgery.

Surgical management of posterior urethral strictures

Primary realignment of disrupted prostatomembranous urethra
Devine has noted that the commoner injury is rupture at the junction of the membranous urethra with the bulb (i.e. below the UG diaphragm). This leaves a competent external urethral sphincter. Many men who are initially impotent after trauma will regain potency within 1–2 years. Causes of impotence include:
- damage to S_{2-4} nerve roots or nerves (anywhere from the posterior pelvis to the prostatic region);
- extensive dissection to control haemorrhage causing damage to sympathetic ganglia and nerves;
- dissection of the posterior and lateral aspects of the prostate, which may cause neural damage;
- damage to the hypogastric or pudendal arteries (needs to be bilateral).

The repair
If the pelvic fracture is displaced and the prostate is still attached the resultant stricture will be very long and difficult to repair. Facilitation of descent of the prostate is brought about by division of the puboprostatic ligaments. These are incised on the anterior aspect of the prostate. This will not increase the incidence of impotence and the prostate will descend to the UG diaphragm once any haematoma has resolved. A suprapubic catheter is inserted. This can all be done by a relatively inexperienced surgeon. If the patient's condition is stable primary realignment may be performed by a more experienced surgeon; it will aid eventual reconstruction.
- Open the bladder at the dome and drain urine.
- Do not dissect pelvic haematoma.
- Palpate the anterior aspect of the prostate and divide puboprostatic ligaments if still intact.

- Put a Foley catheter down the urethra and a second one down the internal urinary meatus and out of the prostatic urethra. Pick up the two ends of the catheters, suture them together and then pull the first Foley up into the bladder.
- The catheter is not put on traction.
- Leave in a suprapubic catheter, close the dome and drain the area of urethral disruption.
- Leave the catheter in for 4 weeks.

This procedure does not prevent a urethral stricture, but does greatly decrease the eventual length of the subsequent stricture, which should then be repaired at 4–6 months.

The role of pubectomy in the repair of membranous strictures
Repair in this way should be undertaken whilst the patient is ambulant, but not within 3 months of the initial injury. This approach has not been favoured previously because of blood loss, but McAninch quotes a mean blood loss of only 800 ml in a series of 30 patients, with a zero incontinence rate (continence depends on an intact bladder neck), 13% restricture rate. A 50% potency rate preoperatively was maintained (all patients were temporarily impotent after the operation, with the longest delay to return of potency being 2 years). All potent patients had normal ejaculation. Advantages of pubectomy:
- improvement of visualization of operative field;
- removal of fistulous tracts and cavities facilitated;
- excision of scar tissue at the prostatic apex facilitated;
- tension free anastomosis.

Perineal repair
Webster has reviewed the incidence of impotence/incontinence after primary realignment; 15 series of 301 patients were managed with primary realignment: 40/201 (20%) were incontinent and 102/252 (44%) were impotent. This contrasted with 236 patients managed by delayed intervention where 4/236 (2%) were incontinent and 26 (11%) were impotent. Webster therefore advocates initial suprapubic cystotomy for tears and complete injury with definitive treatment at 4–6 months. Indications for immediate intervention are:
- injury to bladder neck or rectum;
- massive pelvic haematoma with wide disruption of urethral ends.

Webster performs a delayed one stage urethroplasty through the perineum. Release of the attachment of the bulb to the perineal body is performed. The bulb will tolerate full mobilization as it has a good blood supply. The anterior urethra will survive on collaterals from the corpora and glans. This surgery is contraindicated, however, in patients with previous hypospadias surgery or anterior stricture surgery in whom the blood supply to the anterior urethra may be compromised. A bougie is passed through the suprapubic cystostomy and the proximal urethra identified and fully mobilized. Haematoma is excised rather than incised and both ends of the urethra are spatulated. Anastomosis should be 40 F. If it is not possible to bring both ends of the urethra together then the following are sequentially performed.

1 Further circumferential dissection of the urethra as far as suspensory ligament of penis; will give a further 3 cm.

2 Separate the proximal corporal bodies by 4–5 cm beginning at the crus; there is a 'bloodless' plane between them.

3 Inferior pubectomy: the inferior aspect of the pubis is exposed on dissecting the corpora.

4 Rerouting the urethra around the corporal body; this will give a further 1–2 cm.

Contraindications to this approach are as above plus:

• long strictures
• chronic periurethral cavity sepsis
• rectal, cutaneous and periurethral to bladder base fistulae
• limited access
• previous unsuccessful repair
• incontinence and bladder neck injury.

Further reading

Devine CJ, Jordan GH, Devine PC (1989). Primary realignment of the disrupted prostatomembranous urethra. *Urol Clin North Am*, **16**, 291–295.

McAninch JW (1989). Pubectomy in the repair of membranous urethral strictures. *Urol Clin North Am*, **16**, 297–302.

Webster GD (1983). Prostatomembranous urethral injuries: a review of the literature and a rational approach to their management. *J Urol*, **130**, 898–902.

Webster GD (1989). Perineal repair of membranous urethral stricture. *Urol Clin North Am*, **16**, 303–312.

Management of Renal Trauma

Introduction

Ten per cent of all trauma cases involve the genitourinary tract. This is usually blunt trauma and self-limiting. Five to 10% of blunt and up to

70% of penetrating trauma are major injuries. Major renal injury should be suspected with gross haematuria, shock plus microscopic haematuria, paediatric renal trauma and penetrating renal injuries. In general, minor and limited major injuries are treated conservatively. Unstable major injuries are best treated with prompt surgical exploration as this lessens the risk of continued bleeding, sepsis and renal loss.

Classification
- Minor includes contusion, superficial laceration and self-limiting retroperitoneal bleeds.
- Major includes deep lacerations to the corticomedullary junction, involving the collecting system or major intrarenal vessels.
- Vascular involves complete or partial disruption of the main or segmental arteries or veins.

The mechanism of trauma (blunt or penetrating) is important. Injuries may be staged clinically, radiologically or surgically.
- Common penetrating injuries: knife or gunshot wounds.
- Common blunt injuries: secondary to road traffic accidents, falls, assaults and sport.

Clinical staging
- Microscopic analysis is more reliable in assessing the extent of haemorrhage than dipstick testing.
- Haematuria may be absent in up to 40% of renal injuries and 24% of pedicle injuries.
- Shock plus microscopic haematuria indicates a very high risk group with a likelihood of major vascular injuries (21–25% of cases).
- Penetrating injuries to the flank, abdomen or chest result in renal injury in 6–8% of cases, of which 40–67% will have major vascular injuries.
- Gunshot wounds are particularly difficult to assess clinically due to high incidence of other organ involvement.
- Flank and lumbar wounds are less likely to be associated with other abdominal injuries.
- Patients with no clinical signs who are stable may be treated conservatively.

McAninch has now performed renal exploration in over 200 patients with penetrating injuries and had previously reported major laceration or pedicle injuries in 76% of flank wounds, 81% of anterior abdominal wounds and 40% of lumbar wounds.

Radiological staging

Indications for radiologic assessment
- Penetrating injuries.
- Gross haematuria.
- Shock plus microscopic haematuria.
- Children: the kidneys are much lower and less well protected.
- Intravenous urogram (IVU) is the primary investigation to confirm the presence of a normal contralateral kidney and to assess the extent of the traumatized kidney.

Thirty to 60% of IVU films have been shown to be uninterpretable. Even when abnormal the findings are non-specific. Non-function and extravasation are the only reliable radiologic findings for major and pedicle injuries. A normal IVU and major injury occurs in 20% of cases.

Additional investigations
- Ultrasound scan (USS)
- arteriography
- Computed tomography (CT) scan.

CT scan is now the investigation of choice. It will accurately assess the extent of injury, showing laceration, extravasation, surrounding haemorrhage and vessel injury. CT is both sensitive and specific for perirenal haematoma, parenchymal disruption and extravasation. It also shows associated non-renal injuries and effectively stages renal pedicle injuries. Arterial occlusion is manifest as rim enhancement of the normal renal contour. CT may be improved by contrast enhanced enema which will help to delineate all retroperitoneal structures, in addition to small and large bowel.

Indication for arteriography
- Suspicion of venous injury.
- Indeterminate arterial injury on CT.
- Patients who may require embolization.

Surgical staging and exploration

Indications
- Rarely incomplete staging by clinical and radiologic means.
- Severe urinary extravasation.
- Major vascular injuries with arterial occlusion or significant retroperitoneal haematoma.

Some patients who have not undergone radiology require emergency laparotomy, and some cases of renal trauma will be found unexpectedly during laparotomy. If this occurs then an on-table IVU is mandatory.

- If significant extravasation, non-function, poor opacification or caliceal distortion is found then renal exploration is indicated.
- Failure to explore at this point risks secondary surgery with poor results.
- Expanding or pulsatile haematoma should be explored, but only after vascular control. Vascular occlusion will be required in <20% of patients.

Exploration after trauma
- Blunt trauma: this seldom requires exploration. McAninch reviewed 1193 cases of blunt trauma and only 2.5% required exploration; most other series substantiate this (<10%).
- Penetrating injuries: most penetrating injuries from knife or gunshot wounds require renal exploration.

Absolute indications
- Persistent bleeding: indicates expanding upper retroperitoneal haematoma.
- Pulsatile haematoma: major parenchymal or vessel damage.

Relative indications
- Urinary extravasation: this usually occurs from laceration of the renal pelvis, or parenchymal laceration extending into the collecting system. PUJ avulsion may also occur. Patients with a pre-existing hydronephrosis are more at risk from blunt trauma. Intracapsular extravasation usually subsides spontaneously; extracapsular extravasation may result in a urinoma. If urine is known to be infected, the damaged kidney should be drained.
- Non-viable tissue: parenchymal injury from blunt or penetrating trauma may lead to a large intrarenal haematoma with necrosis. 'Blast' effect from bullets often causes this. If non-viable tissue is left, then abscess formation or hypertension may occur.
- Incomplete staging: some patients require immediate exploration. In such cases perform a one shot IVU on the operating table which establishes the presence of two kidneys. If injured kidney's state is indeterminate, exploration after vascular control is indicated. Initial operation is the best time for repair, delayed operation results in nephrectomy in 50% of cases.

- Arterial thrombosis: blunt trauma may cause main or segmental arterial thrombosis. This needs immediate diagnosis; if more than 12 hours elapse the chance of salvage is remote.

Patients with a delayed diagnosis of main renal artery thrombosis should undergo a nephrectomy if they are having a laparotomy for other reasons. The affected kidney will atrophy and may cause hypertension if not removed. Segmental artery thrombosis is often associated with parenchymal laceration and bleeding, which warrants surgical exploration. If, however, no parenchymal laceration is found, the patient can be treated expectantly as hypertension has not been noted in the long-term.

Operative approach
1 A midline transabdominal approach is preferred with laparotomy for other injuries.
2 Lift the small bowel out of abdomen to expose retroperitoneum.
3 Incise retroperitoneally over the aorta just above the inferior mesenteric artery.
4 If a large haematoma is obscuring the artery make the incision just medial to inferior mesenteric vein.
5 Dissect through the haematoma to the aorta and along it superiorly.
6 Identify the left renal vein; the left and right renal arteries are then easily found.
7 Place vessel loops around the major vessels but do not clamp immediately.

Vascular control has now been established and the kidney can be approached by reflecting the colon. The nephrectomy rate using this method is greatly diminished.

Techniques for reconstruction
Total renal exposure with vascular control is essential; if warm ischaemia time is expected to be more than 1 hour, then ice slush should be used.

- Debridement: remove all non-viable tissue with sharp dissection; active bleeding indicates viability. Preserve the renal capsule for later use. Approximately 30% of one kidney will be sufficient to avoid dialysis.
- Haemostasis: ligate the parenchymal vessels with 4–0 catgut sutures. Do not use non-absorbable sutures. Large veins coursing through the parenchyma can be tied (there are good intrarenal venous collaterals). Segmental or interlobar artery ligation will cause

parenchymal infarction, so use absorbable collagen for haemostasis.
- Collecting system closure: this must be watertight; use a 4–0 running absorbable suture.
- Defect coverage:
renal capsule
pedicle omental graft
free peritoneal graft.
These will all prevent extravasation.

Partial nephrectomy
Indicated for extensively damaged lower or upper poles, this needs full exposure and vascular control. Suture ligate individual vessels and use as above for defect coverage.

Renorraphy
This technique is employed when the midportion of the kidney is damaged. All non-viable tissue should be excised, the collecting system closed and parenchymal margins approximated. Sutures are placed over an absorbable gelatin sponge bolster. If parenchymal margins cannot be brought together a pedicled omental graft or absorbable mesh should be used.

Vascular injuries
- Blunt trauma causes vessel thrombosis, rarely haemorrhage.
- Main veins should be repaired with a 5 or 6–0 vascular suture, after clamping renal artery.
- Injured segmental veins may be safely ligated.
- Vascular injuries are usually associated with damage to other major organs including: liver, spleen, small bowel, colon, stomach.
- Deaths are usually related to other injuries and not renal injuries.
- Ninety per cent of pedicle injuries occur in children and young adults, 75% of patients are male.
- Major pedicle injuries occur most commonly with blunt trauma; penetrating trauma accounts for only 4–24% of injuries (L > R (X2), bilateral 5%, artery 70%, vein 20%, both 10%).
- The mortality rate with pedicle injury is 40%, usually due to other injuries.
- Pedicle injuries are acceleration/deceleration injuries which cause intimal tears followed by subintimal dissection and thrombosis. More severe injuries may rupture the muscularis and adventitia.

Further reading

McAninch JW, Carroll PR (1989). Renal exploration after trauma. *Urol Clin North Am*, **16**, 203–212.

McAninch JW, Carroll PR (1982). Renal trauma: kidney preservation through improved vascular control—a refined approach. *J Trauma*, **22**, 285–289.

Cass AS (1989). Renovascular injuries from external trauma. Diagnosis, treatment and outcome. *Urol Clin North Am*, **16**, 213–220.

Sandler CM, Toombs BD (1981). Computed tomographic evaluation of blunt renal injuries. *Radiology*, **141**, 461.

McAninch JW, Carroll PR, Klosterman PW *et al.* (1991). Renal reconstruction after injury. *J Urol*, **145**, 932–937.

Continent Catheterizable Pouches

Introduction

The two main principles involved in pouch formation are to attempt a spherical configuration and to disrupt peristaltic bowel activity. The two favoured sites for a continent stoma are the umbilicus, and bikini line in the lower quadrant through the rectus bulge. The former is used for wheelchair patients, the latter for ambulant young men and women. There are also orthotopic locations for catheterizable portals, e.g. construction of neourethra in introitus of females. Intussuscepted nipple valves are not easy to self-catheterize in an orthotopic position, but imbricated or tapered ileal segments are. The most technically demanding feature of each pouch construction is the continence mechanism.

Formation of a catheterizable continence zone

Appendiceal tunnelling

The technique is similar to that used for ureterocolonic anastomosis; the main problems are:

- the appendix may be absent;
- the appendix may be too short to permit tunnelling and to reach the abdominal wall.

    There are two methods of using the appendix (Mitrofanoff principle):

- excision of appendix and button of caecum, reversing it and tunnelled re-implantation (Duckett & Snyder);
- appendix left in continuity, folded cephalad and buried in a caecal tunnel (Riedmiller *et al.*).

Ileal mechanisms

- Imbricated terminal ileum is suitable for all pouches when using an ileocaecal segment. It forms a good continence mechanism, but the ileal neourethra may lengthen with time. One criticism is loss of the ileocaecal valve.
- Intussuscepted ileal nipple valve: this is the most demanding technically; there is a significant learning curve and the stability of the Kock nipple valve is disappointing in a significant number of patients (10–15%). Stability improved by:
  removal of mesenteric attachments from middle 6–8 cm of bowel used for valve;
  fixation of pouch and nipple valve together by a variety of suturing and stapling methods.
  Stones form on exposed staples.
  Initial capacities of gastric and Kock pouches are 150 ml, right colonic pouches 300 ml. All patients with pouches will have bacteriuria, but should only be treated if symptomatic.
- Urinary retention is uncommon and is usually related to nipple valves. This should be treated as an emergency.
- Recatheterization may sometimes need either fluoroscopy or flexible cystoscopy.
- Intraperitoneal rupture of pouches has been reported; it is more common in neurological patients and is associated with mild abdominal trauma. Treatment is with immediate pouch decompression and abdominal exploration if patient has an acute abdomen; otherwise catheter drainage and antibiotics will suffice.

Different pouches

Kock continent ileal reservoir (Kock 1982; Skinner 1987)

- Uses 70–80 cm of terminal ileum.
- Nipple valve continence mechanism, stabilized by stapling to pouch, and absorbable mesh collar.
- Complications are usually specific to the nipple valve: (i) fistulae due to pinhole from stapling device, (ii) prolapse of nipple valve, (iii) shortening of nipple valve secondary to ischaemia.
- Failure rate of the valve is 15% in the best of hands. Kock's original series reports an 80% reoperation rate, others 30%.

Mainz pouch

- Terminal ileum and right colon; the ileocaecal valve is used to stabilize the nipple valve.

- Uses 15 cm of caecum and ascending colon and two equal sized limbs of terminal ileum (2×15cm) for the pouch and a further 20cm of ileum for the nipple valve. Initial capacities are higher than the Kock pouch.
- Stabilization of nipple valve by the ileocaecal valve results in a negligible revision rate.

Right colon pouches with intussuscepted terminal ileum
The terminal ileum is intussuscepted through the ileocaecal valve. These are all variations on the Mansson reservoir.
- UCLA pouch (Raz).
- Duke pouch (Webster).
- LeBag (Light and Scardino).

The only real difference between them is in the construction of the continent nipple valve.

UCLA
Fifteen cm of distal ileum is used for the intussusception. This is fixed through the ileocaecal valve after the caecum has been opened along its anterior taenia using a bladeless GIA stapling device. Capacities: 600–700 ml; 88% dry by day and night.

Duke
A similar length of bowel is intussuscepted and brought through the ileocaecal valve, but fixed to back wall of pouch by suture rather than staple device (thus no foreign bodies or stone formation).

LeBag
A similar configuration to the LeBag orthotopic bladder, but extra distal ileum is used for the intussuscepted nipple valve.

Indiana pouch (also Miami and Florida)
Eponym used depends on reconfiguration of bowel.
- The use of a double imbricating suture is employed to strengthen the ileocaecal valve; the rest of the terminal ileum is tapered (Benjay & Politano 1988).
- Right colon is used for the pouch.
- Indiana pouch: average capacity 400–500 ml; continence rate 93%; high peak contractions (47 cm H_2O).
- Miami pouch: average capacity 750 ml; maximum pressure 20 cm H_2O.
- Florida pouch: average capacity 400–1200 ml; pressures 18–55 cm H_2O.
- Hyperchloraemia in 70% of patients; 7.2% reoperation rate.

Sigmoid pouches used mainly in USA and Egypt, either partially or totally detubularized.

Advantages
- Easily brought down to membranous urethra.
- Loss of sigmoid colon has no nutritional impact or effect on bowel function.

Disadvantages
- Sigmoid often affected by diverticular disease and malignancy.
- Capacities around 750 ml at <20 cm H_2O pressure.

Further reading

Duckett JW, Snyder HM III (1987). The Mitrofanoff principle in continent urinary reservoirs. *Semin Urol*, **5**, 55–62.

Reidmiller H, Steinbach F, Thuroff J *et al.* (1990). Continent appendix stoma, a modification of the MAINZ pouch technique. *EUA congress, Amsterdam, June 1990.*

Kock NG, Nilson AE, Nilsson LO *et al.* (1982). Urinary diversion via a continent ileal reservoir. Clinical results in 12 patients. *J Urol*, **128**, 469–475.

Skinner DG, Lieskovsky G, Boyd S (1987). Continuing experience with the continent ileal reservoir (Kock) as an alternative to cutaneous urinary diversion: an update after 250 cases. *J Urol*, **141**, 1140–1145.

Benjay DE, Politano VA (1988). A stapled and nonstapled tapered distal ileum for construction of a continent colonic reservoir. *J Urol*, **140**, 491–494.

Urodynamic Data on Pouches Used for Orthotopic Bladders (Table 3, p. 72)

Further reading

Camey M, LeDuc A (1979). L'entérocystoplastie après cystoprostatectomie totale pour cancer de la vessie. *Ann Urol*, **13**, 114–123.

Mansson W, Colleen S (1990). Experience with a detubularized right colonic segment for bladder replacement. *Scand J Urol Nephrol*, **24**, 53–56.

Goldwasser B, Benson RC, Jr (1986). Continent urinary diversion. *Mayo Clin Proc*, **61**, 615–621.

Light JK, Scardino PT (1986). Radical cystectomy with preservation of sexual and urinary function: use of the ileocolonic pouch ('LeBag'). *Urol Clin North Am*, **13**, 261–270.

Studer UE, Speigel T, Cassonova GA *et al.* (1991). Ileal bladder substitute: antireflux nipple or afferent tubular segment? *Eur Urol*, **20**, 315–326.

Table 3 Urodynamic data on pouches used for orthotopic bladders

	Daytime continence	Night-time continence	Basal pouch pressure (cm H$_2$O)	Max pouch pressure (cm H$_2$O)	Mean pouch capacity (>6/12)
Camey II 1990 (65cm ileum)	96%	75%	10	30	434 ml
Vesica Ileale Padovana 1990 (Jelly roll)	92%	87%	3–5	10–30	400–600 ml
Ulm 1988 (Ileal Neobladder)	82%	82%	10	26	775 ml
Orthotopic hemi-Kock 1987 (Ileum)	88%	88%	20	20	300–750 ml
Studer pouch (hemi-Kock variant) 1988 (Ileum)	100%	50%	N/K	20–35	450 ml
Mainz pouch 1985 (Ileocaecal)	93%	75%	33	41	510 ml
LeBag 1986 (ileocaecal)	85%	85%	N/K	20–58	400–700 ml
Goldwasser and Benson; Mayo Clinic 1986 (Right colonic segments)	N/K	N/K	N/K	44	N/K
Mansson pouch 1990	100%	N/K	11	22	320–600 ml

N/K = Not Known

Standardization of Terminology Used in the Description of Intestinal Urinary Reservoirs

Bladder augmentation
This increases bladder capacity and may be performed in several ways.
- Autoaugmentation, without the use of other tissues.
- By the use of other tissues (e.g. small bowel enterocystoplasty, large bowel intestinocystoplasty, stomach gastrocystoplasty) being incorporated into the bladder—the bladder may or may not be partially resected, and the bowel may or may not be reconfigured or detubularized.

Bladder substitution
The bladder is replaced *in situ* by other tissues such as intestine, which has been detubularized and reconfigured; this is known as an orthotopic bladder substitution.
- Total substitution: all the bladder, including the bladder neck in females and the bladder neck and prostate in males is removed.
- Subtotal substitution: the intestinal reservoir is anastamosed to the bladder neck following subtotal excision of the bladder. The procedure is usually performed for benign conditions such as interstitial cystitis.

Anastomosis of reservoir to outlet
- The reservoir may be anastomosed to the native urethra.
- The reservoir may be anastomosed to the native urethra supported by an artificial urinary sphincter/sling to aid continence.
- The reservoir may be anastomosed to a urethral substitute (usually a small section of reconfigured bowel) in the native (orthotopic) urethral position.

Continent cutaneous urinary diversion
An intestinal pouch forms the urinary reservoir, with a continence mechanism extending from the pouch wall to a heterotopically placed outlet—usually a cutaneous stoma placed either at the umbilicus or below the bikini line. Tissues used for the continence mechanism include:
- appendix
- imbricated and tapered small bowel.

Continent anal urinary diversion

A reservoir fashioned from bowel, either in continuity or isolated, using the anal sphincter as a continent outlet.

Further reading

Thuroff JW, Mattiasson A, Andersen JT *et al.* (1996). The standardization of terminology and assessment of functional characteristics of intestinal urinary reservoirs. *Br J Urol,* **78**, 516–523.

Hinman F, Jr (1988). Selection of intestinal segments for bladder substitution: physical and physiological characteristics. *J Urol,* **139**, 519–523.

Woodhouse CRJ (1992). Lower urinary tract reconstruction in young patients. *Br J Urol,* **70**, 113–120.

Hendry WF (1996). Bladder replacement by ileocystoplasty after cystectomy for cancer: comparison of two techniques. *Br J Urol,* **78**, 74–79.

Urodynamics

Bladder Outflow Obstruction

Introduction

Seventy per cent of men over the age of 70 years have BPH but only 10–20% will undergo prostatectomy. The early results of operation are unsatisfactory in 25% of men. This is partly because detrusor instability occurs in 70% of men presenting with bladder outflow obstruction, which will only resolve in 70–75% of patients following relief of obstruction. A symptomatic diagnosis of bladder outflow obstruction does not always correlate with a urodynamic diagnosis or with clinical estimation of the size of the prostate gland.

Unsatisfactory outcome from operation is associated with:
- preoperative symptoms of urge incontinence;
- small prostatic size and resected weight;
- low voiding pressures and low urethral resistance.

Flow rates

- Should include observation of maximal flow rate (Q_{max}, ml/s).
- Pattern and voided volume.
- Voided volumes of less than 150 ml may lead to erroneous results.
- Patients often improve performance on repeated flows.
- There is considerable overlap between patients with and without symptoms of obstruction.

Abrams and Griffiths classified the risk of bladder outflow obstruction according to flow rate.
- The probability that a patient with $Q_{max} < 10$ ml/s is obstructed is 88%.
- The probability that a patient with $Q_{max} > 15$ ml/s is not obstructed is 68%.
- Pressure–flow studies are recommended for patients in the equivocal range.

Pressure–flow studies

These were first described by Refisch in 1897. Bladder and intra-abdominal pressure (usually rectal) are measured simultaneously.
- Intra-abdominal pressure is subtracted from the bladder pressure to give detrusor pressure.

- Measurement is via fluid filled lines with transducer levelled at pubic symphysis, or more recently solid-state transducer tipped catheters (non-fluid filled).
- Detrusor pressure must be synchronized by correcting for delay in flow rate measurement.

Most UK centres use urethral lines for bladder pressure measurement and for filling. Some investigators remove the urethral filling line for the voiding phase. Many European countries routinely use suprapubic lines.

- Low pressure, high flow is considered unobstructed.
- High pressure, low flow is considered obstructed.
- Patients falling between these criteria form an equivocal group in whom urodynamic diagnosis can be difficult.

Nomograms for plots of pressure and flow

The Abrams–Griffiths nomogram
This classifies patients into the following groups:
- obstructed
- non-obstructed
- equivocal.

Equivocal cases can be further classified by plotting a curve connecting pressure–flow values throughout micturition. If the mean slope of the subsequent plot is > 2 cm H_2O/ml/s or the closing pressure > 40 cm H_2O then the plot is considered obstructed.

Linearized passive urethral resistance relation (Schafer nomogram)
This nomogram is derived from Schafer's passive urethral resistance relation (PURR) where a parabolic curve fitted to the pressure–flow plot determines the detrusor pressure at minimum flow (i.e. opening pressure) and defines urethral resistance. The pressure–flow plot is divided into seven bands (O–VII) and grades the degree of obstruction.

Group specific urethral resistance factor
Group specific urethral resistance factor (URA) is calculated from Q_{max} and P_{det} at Q_{max} via a standard formula. This provides a single value expressed in cm H_2O. Values greater than 29 cm H_2O are considered to be obstructed.

Detrusor contraction strength
Detrusor contraction strength (WF) is a measure of the work done by

the contracting detrusor, related to the velocity of shortening of the detrusor fibres. It is calculated by computer throughout the voiding cycle and requires the residual urine value.

Further reading
Abrams PH, Griffiths DJ (1979). The assessment of prostatic obstruction from urodynamic measurements and from residual urine. *Br J Urol*, **51**, 129–134.

Griffiths DJ, Van Mastrigt R, Bosch R (1989). Quantification of urethral resistance and bladder function during voiding, with special reference to the effects of prostate size reduction on urethral obstruction due to benign prostatic hyperplasia. *Neurourol Urodynam*, **8**, 17–27.

Griffiths DJ (1977) Urodynamic assessment of bladder function. *Br J Urol*, **49**, 29–36.

Neal DE, Styles RA, Ng T, Powell PH, Thong J, Ramsden PD (1987). Relationship between voiding pressures, symptoms and urodynamic findings in 253 men undergoing prostatectomy. *Br J Urol*, **60**, 554–559.

Neal DE, Ramsden PD, Sharples L *et al.* (1989). Outcome of elective prostatectomy. *Br Med J*, **299**, 762–767.

Schafer W (1985). Urethral resistance? Urodynamic concepts of physiological and pathological bladder outlet function during voiding. *Neurourol Urodynam*, **4**, 161–201.

Turner-Warwick R (1979). Observations on the function and dysfunction of the sphincter and detrusor mechanisms. *Urol Clin North Am*, **6**, 13–30.

Residual Urine

Definition
The volume of urine remaining in the bladder immediately following the completion of micturition.

- It is important to establish the time between voiding and measurement.
- An artificially elevated residual urine may result from voiding in unfamiliar surroundings, to command or with an overfilled bladder.
- An isolated finding of a significant residual urine should be confirmed.
- Careful interpretation is required in the presence of vesicoureteric reflux or bladder diverticula.
- The absence of residual urine does not exclude bladder outflow obstruction or dysfunction.

Assessment
- Drainage: invasive and incomplete in up to 26% of cases.
- IVU: inaccurate but useful if zero.

- Real time ultrasound: accuracy ± 10–25% for bladder volumes over 100 ml; worse for smaller volumes; safe and non-invasive.

Ultrasound images the bladder transabdominally in the transverse and sagittal planes. Volume is calculated as $0.52 \times$ height $\times$ width $\times$ anteroposterior diameter.

Significance of residual urine

- Residual urine is a common finding in men with symptoms of bladder outflow obstruction.
- Ten per cent of such men will develop acute retention over a 7 year period.
- A residual urine of >50 ml may be found in 50% of patients with prostatic symptoms who have no urodynamic obstruction.
- Large residual volumes are a feature of detrusor failure.
- Eighty-five per cent of healthy females under 55 years have small residuals.
- Healthy elderly men have been shown to have small residuals (mean $= 28$ ml, max $= 100$ ml).
- Residual urine volumes >300ml are associated with the development of upper tract dilatation and chronic renal failure, particularly in the presence of elevated detrusor pressures (Abrams 1979; Styles 1986).
- Residual urine is shown to decrease after prostatectomy.
- There is no correlation between preoperative residual urine and postoperative success rate.
- Men with residual volumes >300 ml and a pressure rise during filling of >25 cm H_2O, known to be at risk of upper tract dilatation, do well after prostatectomy with resolution of upper tract dilatation and improved bladder emptying.

Further reading

Abrams PH, Dunn M, George NJR (1978). Urodynamic findings in chronic retention of urine and their relevance to the results of surgery. *Br Med J*, **2**, 1258–1260.

Andersen JT, Jacobsen O, Worm-Petersen J, Hald T (1978). Bladder function in healthy elderly males. *Scand J Urol Nephrol*, **12**, 123–127.

Styles RA, Ramsden PD, Neal DE (1986). Chronic retention of urine: the relationship between upper tract dilatation and bladder pressure. *Br J Urol*, **58**, 647–651.

Styles RA, Ramsden PD, Neal DE (1991). The outcome of prostatectomy on chronic retention of urine. *J Urol*, **146**, 1029–1033.

Ambulatory Urodynamics

Introduction

Ambulatory urodynamic monitoring (AM) is an established clinical investigation of detrusor function. Conventional artificial filling cystometry (CMG) is restricted by:

- the artificial speed of filling
- non-physiological filling media at non-body temperature
- restricted mobility
- hostile surroundings
- 'command performance'
- invasive monitoring and filling lines.

AM systems currently use fine urethral catheters but allow free mobility and do not restrict the patient to the examination room. Several commercial systems available (e.g. Gaeltec, Dantec, Weiss). The Freeman 'Urolog' system has been described in the literature.

- All systems use a portable recorder which collects digitized information from bladder and rectal lines.
- Urolog uses solid state Gaeltec catheters (6F) which are comfortable, easy to use and reliable.
- The pressure transducer is in the tip and connected by wire through the catheter to the recorder.
- The pressure transducers are calibrated before every study.
- Urolog was one of the first systems to quantitatively measure urinary leakage, by means of a resistance strip built into an absorbent disposable nappy.

Some systems use water filled lines, but the recorder transducer must be situated at the pubic symphysis (water filled lines are cheap and disposable).

Detrusor instability

- Ambulatory manometry is significantly more sensitive in detecting detrusor instability than conventional CMG; this has been shown in all published studies.
- Sixty per cent of patients diagnosed with detrusor instability on AM have previously normal CMGs.
- Thirty-eight per cent of healthy volunteers have been shown to be unstable on AM compared to 17% with CMG filling at 50 ml/min, and zero with CMG at 100 ml/min.

Neuropathic bladder

Webb and Styles (1989) examined patients with neurogenic bladder dysfunction. Spontaneous detrusor contractions were found more frequently with AM, but the frequency of these contractions correlated positively with the poor compliance (high filling pressures) seen during CMG, whilst filling pressures were significantly lower during AM. Those patients with upper tract dilatation were found to have greater residual volumes and higher pressure rises during CMG with more frequent phasic activity during AM.

Chronic retention

Styles examined men with chronic urinary retention (1986, 1987).

- Poor detrusor compliance found during CMG was not found on AM.
- Previously unreported phasic activity was seen during AM which correlated to both the development of upper tract dilatation and to the poor compliance seen during CMG.

In general

- During AM, residual volumes, pressure rises during filling and voided volumes are lower than in conventional CMG; however, maximum voiding pressures are significantly higher in AM.
- Phasic activity is more easily detected and is seen to be more frequent and of greater amplitude on AM.

Standardization

Standardized terminology for urodynamic investigation is devised by the International Continence Society Committee on Standardization of Terminology (Table 4).

Further reading

Abrams P, Blaivas JG, Stanton SL, Andersen JT (1988). The standardisation of terminology of lower urinary tract function. The ICS Committee on Standardisation of Terminology. *Scand J Urol Nephrol*, **114**, (Suppl.) 5–19.

Styles RA, Neal DE, Ramsden PD (1986). Comparison of long-term monitoring and standard cystometry in chronic retention of urine. *Br J Urol*, **58**, 652–656.

Styles RA, Neal DE, Griffiths CJ *et al.* (1987). Long-term monitoring of the bladder in chronic retention: phasic activity and upper tract dilatation. *Neurourol Urodynam*, **6**, 223–224.

Robertson AS, Griffiths CJ, Ramsden PD, Neal DE (1994). Bladder function in healthy volunteers: ambulatory monitoring and conventional urodynamic studies. *Br J Urol*, **73**, 242–249.

Webb RJ, Styles RA, Griffiths CJ, Ramsden PD, Neal DE (1989). Ambulatory

monitoring of bladder pressures in patients with low compliance as a result of neurogenic bladder dysfunction. *Br J Urol*, **64**, 150–154.
Webb RJ, Griffiths CJ, Ramsden PD, Neal DE (1990). Measurement of voiding

Table 4 Standard definitions for urodynamic investigation.

Premicturition pressure	The pressure recorded immediately before the initial isovolumetric contraction.
Opening pressure	The pressure at the onset of flow.
Maximum pressure	The maximum measured pressure.
Pressure at maximum flow	The pressure recorded at maximum flow rate.
Contraction pressure at maximum flow	The difference between pressure at maximum flow and premicturition pressure.
Maximum cystometric capacity	The volume at which the patient has a strong desire to void, or at which leakage occurs.
Effective cystometric capacity	Maximum cystometric capacity minus residual urine.
Functional bladder capacity	Assessed from frequency volume chart.
Total bladder capacity	Maximal functional bladder capacity plus residual urine.
Detrusor/sphincter dyssynergia	Detrusor contraction concurrent with an inappropriate contraction of the urethral and/or periurethral striated muscle.
Detrusor/bladder neck dyssynergia	Detrusor contraction concurrent with an objectively demonstrated failure of bladder neck opening.
The unstable detrusor	This is one that is shown objectively to contract, spontaneously or on provocation, during the filling phase whilst the patient is attempting to inhibit micturition.
Detrusor hyperreflexia	Overactivity due to disturbance of nervous control mechanisms, and should be confirmed by objective evidence of a neurological disorder.

pressures on ambulatory monitoring: comparison with conventional cystometry. *Br J Urol*, **65**, 152–154.

Webb RJ, Ramsden PD, Neal DE (1991). Ambulatory monitoring and electronic measurement of urinary leakage in the diagnosis of detrusor instability and incontinence. *Br J Urol*, **68**, 148–152.

Whitaker Test

Indication

Devised to diagnose and quantify obstruction in the upper urinary tract. Interpretation of the result is often difficult.

Methodology

Access to the upper urinary tract is obtained via percutaneous nephrostomy puncture. Pressure is measured in the renal pelvis and in the bladder whilst saline (or contrast medium) is infused into the proximal upper urinary tract at rates of 5–20 ml/min. The pressure gradient across the suspected obstruction is measured. If obstructed then a rising pressure will be seen, dependent on the flow rate and the distension of the system. In unobstructed cases the system will tolerate a high flow with little or no pressure rise.

- Pressure stabilization of less than $10\,cm\,H_2O$ is considered unobstructed.
- Pressures greater than $20\,cm\,H_2O$ are obstructed.

Further reading

Whitaker RH (1973). Methods of assessing obstruction in dilated ureters. *Br J Urol*, **45**, 15–22.

Renal Transplantation

Patient Management prior to Transplantation

Access

Good access is required to permit optimal flow (180–300 ml/min) to achieve efficient dialysis. Clotting, stenosis and infection are the bane of access sites. Around 40–90% of septicaemic episodes in patients on dialysis originate from access sites.

Access routes

Percutaneous double lumen cannula

These are useful for immediate or temporary cannulation and while waiting for maturation of an arterio-venous (AV) fistula. They can be used for months by rotating sites.

- Femoral vein: makes ambulation difficult, but easier to perform.
- Subclavian vein: complications which can occur are arterial puncture, haemothorax, SVC perforation, pneumothorax, vein thrombosis and phlebitis, late stenosis.

Shunts

Give high blood flow but have limited life span and high risk of infection. These are rarely used and are less desirable for chronic renal failure (CRF).

- Quinton–Scribner shunt: connects a prosthesis between the distal radial artery and forearm vein.
- Thomas shunt: femoral artery–femoral vein shunt.
- Posterior tibial artery–saphenous vein shunt.

Fistula

- Primary: direct or using saphenous vein for interposition.
- Secondary: at the same sites using PTFE or Dacron.

Types of fistula

- Brescia–Cimino fistula: radial artery to cephalic vein.
- Ulnar artery to cephalic vein.
- Brachial artery to cephalic vein.
  The AV fistula is superior to the shunt, and a native vein fistula is

preferable to a secondary prosthetic fistula. Fistulae may be difficult to create because of atherosclerotic vessels, poor superficial veins or most often due to fibrosis of veins secondary to repeated intravenous infusions and blood sampling.

In preparation for treatment of end stage renal disease (ESRD), preservation of extremity veins and early placement of an AV fistula to allow time for maturation (which takes several months) is good practice. Elbow fistulae have better long-term patency than forearm ones. The principles of 'distal before proximal' and 'autogenous before prosthetic' holds good for adults as it does for children.

Fistulae can result in aneurysm formation, thrombosis, congestive heart failure and infection. Efficiency of dialysis may be reduced with compromised flow in a fistula.

Diet
Dietary manipulation can slow down progression of renal failure. Protein restriction on its own or in combination with phosphorus restriction are the usual dietary modifications. Adequate intake of calories and vitamins must be maintained. However, these diets are less important once established on a maintenance dialysis programme.

Anaemia
Erythropoietin levels in renal failure and when on dialysis have been reported to be low. However, in those with polycystic disease or cyst development, when on long-term dialysis levels are higher.

Occult gastrointestinal (GI) losses are high in dialysis-dependent patients. Other sources of loss are in dialysers and lines, mechanical due to the pumps, blood sampling and dietary deficiencies.

Low erythropoietin levels are also seen after bilateral nephrectomy, aluminium toxicity and hypertransfusion which suppresses erythropoiesis.

Management
- Transfusions should be restricted, apart from those on erythropoietin, and be used for severe acute loss only as they have other complications.
- Efficient dialysis has been shown to improve erythropoiesis and reduce losses in lines and dialysers.
- Maintenance of iron stores by oral supplementation, and also folate and vitamin supplements.
- Androgens are used in those who cannot receive erythropoietin.
- Human recombinant erythropoietin (rHuEPO) replacement therapy.
  Uncontrolled hypertension is a contraindication for therapy. rHuEPO is given at 110–120 U/kg in 2–3 doses intravenously or subcutaneously

following dialysis. Patients tend to become iron deficient with rHuEPO therapy. They need regular monitoring of iron status by measurement of serum ferritin and transferrin saturation, and iron supplements.

Further reading

Kjellstrand CM (1978). The Achilles' heel of the hemodialysis patient. *Arch Intern Med*, **138**, 1063–1064.

Lumsden AB, MacDonald MJ, Allen RC, Dodson TF (1994). Hemodialysis access in the paediatric patient population. *Am J Surg*, **168**, 197–201.

Frohling PT, Krupki F, Kokot F, Vetter K, Kaschube I, Lindenau K (1989). What are the most important factors in the progression of renal failure? *Kidney Int*, **36** (Suppl. 27), 106–109.

de Klerk G, Wilmink JM, Rosengarten PC, Vet RJ, Goudsmit R (1982). Serum erythropoietin (ESF) titres in anaemia of chronic renal failure. *J Lab Clin Med*, **100**, 720–734.

Ireland R, Lutkin J, Evans R *et al.* (1982). Blood losses from patients on chronic haemodialysis. *Dial Transplant*, **11**, 782–784.

Macdougall IC (1995). How to get the best out of rHuEPO. *Nephrol Dial Transplant*, **10** (Suppl. 2), 85–91.

Fertility and Reproductive Issues

Introduction

Uraemia is an effective contraceptive. Transplantation usually results in return of normal function with resumption of menstruation, ovulation and conception. The incidence of spontaneous first trimester abortion is 16%, and 22% have therapeutic abortion. Of those pregnancies that progress beyond this, 92% end successfully.

Risks

- Conception and the outcome of continuing with the pregnancy depend on multiple factors. If the serum creatinine is over 132 μmol/l (1.5 mg/dl) the risks are high. The kidney is unlikely to be able to adequately respond to the demands of pregnancy and the glomerular filtration rate (GFR) cannot rise further.

- In non-transplant individuals the presence of hypertension prior to conception increases the incidence of maternal and fetal complications. Thirty per cent of pregnancies after a transplant are complicated by hypertension and one-third will develop pre-eclampsia.

- Asymptomatic bacteriuria is no more common than in normal pregnancy or in non-pregnant recipients. Overt urinary tract infection occurs in about 25–40% of normal pregnancies. It is unlikey that this will be less in the pregnant recipient.

Recommendations/preconception counselling
- Live donor kidney recipients should wait for at least 1 year and others for 2 years, as the risk of rejection is highest until then.
- Hypertension should be easily managed or none at all.
- Stable renal function. Serum creatinine less than 132 µmol/l or 1.5 mg/dl.
- No rejection, proteinuria, pelvicalyceal distension.
- Maintained on less than 15 mg/day of Prednisolone and 2 mg/kg/day of Azathioprine. Cyclosporin is probably best avoided, though safe doses are quoted to be 5 mg/kg/day.

Maternal complications and management
- Complications include steroid induced hypertension, leucopenia, septicaemia, rejection and uterine rupture. Permanent reduction in renal function occurs in 15% of cases.
- The risk of the allograft obstructing labour is remote, although has been reported, and caesarean section is therefore not mandatory.
- Ureteric obstruction is also unusual.
- Rejection episodes are no more common during pregnancy and often occur after child birth.
- Augmentation of steroids during labour.
- Prophylactic antibiotics to be used before any procedure.

Fetal complications and management
- In the fetus, prematurity, respiratory distress syndrome, intrauterine growth retardation, congenital anomalies and infections have been reported. Sixty per cent are preterm and small for gestational age.
- Immunosuppressives affect the fetus more than the mother. Patients should be on lowest possible doses of Prednisolone and Azathioprine.
- Cyclosporin has been reported to cause growth retardation and affect fetal renal function.
- Cyclosporin levels in breast milk are higher than blood levels. Breast feeding is to be avoided.
- Long-term monitoring of children needed as the sequelae with respect to malignancies and the next generation are not known.

Contraceptive counselling
- Sterilization at the time of transplantation if the couple have no desire for any further children.
- Avoid Intrauterine Contraceptive Device in view of the risk of infection.

- Diaphragm or low dose oral contraceptive. The risk of hypertension or thromboembolic disease is increased with the latter. There is also the risk of drug interaction with Cyclosporin.

Male factors
- Dialysis-dependent patients have diminished libido and spermatogenesis; transplantation reverses both.
- Male fertility is at greater risk from the surgical procedure; ligation of the spermatic cord is to be avoided in those still planning to have children.
- Use of one internal iliac artery may be safe, but if a second transplant is required the external iliac artery should be used to prevent impotence.

Further reading
Lindheimer MD, Katz AI (1991). The kidney and hypertension in pregnancy. In: *The Kidney*, Vol. 2, (eds BM Brenner, FC Rector), 4th edn, pp. 1551–1595. Saunders, Philadelphia.

Surian M, Imbasciati E, Cosci P *et al.* (1984). Glomerular disease and pregnancy. A study of 123 pregnancies in patients with primary and secondary glomerular diseases. *Nephron*, **36**, 101–105.

Davison JM (1995). Towards long-term graft survival in renal transplantation: pregnancy. *Nephrol Dial Transplant*, **10** (Suppl. 1), 85–89.

Davison JM (1987). Pregnancy in renal allograft recipients. Prognosis and management. *Clin Obst Gynaecol*, **1**, 1027–1045.

Immunosuppression

Introduction
Immunosuppression (IS) aims to prevent or reverse rejection episodes. The drugs commonly used, Azathioprine (Aza), Prednisolone (Pred) and Cyclosporin A (CsA), try to block T-cell proliferation at different sites in an effort to prevent rejection. Steroids are also used in the treatment of acute rejection.

Azathioprine
- Useful for inhibiting primary immune responses. It blocks T-cell activation at the most distal point, and acts by blocking DNA and RNA synthesis.
- Suppresses the number of circulating monocytes capable of differentiating into macrophages.
- Less useful in reversal of acute rejection. As it is metabolized in the liver its dose need not be reduced in rejection.

Side effects

The major one is myelotoxicity with leucocytes more affected than platelets. GI toxicity, hepatotoxicity, alopecia and risk of neoplasia (especially cutaneous).

New antimetabolites: mizoribine, RS61443, brequinar sodium, leflunomide.

Corticosteroids

* Steroids are used in conjunction with one of the other agents. Steroids block the T-cell activation cascade at the most proximal point by blocking activation of IL-1 and IL-6.
* In high doses their effect on macrophage function alters the effector phase of graft rejection.

Side effects

Apart from the usual Cushingoid appearance, those which have a major influence on the transplantee are growth retardation in children, impaired wound healing, hypertension, diabetes and avascular necrosis of bone.

Cyclosporin A

* This is a fungal decapeptide. CsA inhibits IL-2 induction which is critical to the T-cell cascade. It is most useful as preventive therapy.
* Peak concentration occurs 2–4 hours after oral therapy. As bioavailability is so variable and there is such a narrow range between immunosuppressive and toxic doses, blood level monitoring is recommended. Monitoring is complicated by many variables such as haematocrit, temperature, assay method.
* CsA is metabolized in the liver by the P-450 microsomal enzyme system, by virtue of which there are significant drug interactions. Erythromycin, Ketoconazole, Diltiazem, oral contraceptives and Metoclopramide are among those that increase CsA levels while Phenobarbitone, Phenytoin, Carbamazepine, Rifampicin and Izoniazid decrease CsA levels.

Side effects

The most common one is nephrotoxicity. CsA has a vasoconstrictive effect on the afferent glomerular arterioles associated with increased vascular resistance, stimulation of the sympathetic system and rennin–angiotensin system, and synthesis of the vasoconstrictor thromboxane. It is also a tubular toxin and causes interstitial fibrosis. Acute nephrotoxicity can occur after the first dose. The functional toxicity of CsA with postischaemic renal damage, seen in the immediate post-transplant situation, may be additive to produce oliguria.

CsA toxicity usually presents as non-oliguric renal dysfunction with elevated serum creatinine. This form of renal dysfunction can also occur in rejection. Because those on CsA can present without fever or tenderness, no pathognomonic laboratory or clinical parameter can reliably distinguish between CsA nephrotoxicity and allograft rejection. The diagnosis is based on exclusion, response to CsA dose reduction or a biopsy. The two can occur simultaneously. Other side effects include hepatotoxicity, diabetes, neuropathy, tremor, gingival hypertrophy and hypertrichosis.

New anti T-cell agents: Rapamicin, FK506 (Tacrolimus), Cyclosporin neoral.

Polyclonal immunoglobulins

Antilymphocyte globulin (ALG) and antithymocyte globulin (ATG) have been available since the 1970s and have been more effective than steroids in reversing rejection. Cultured lymphoblasts free of contaminating blood cells are used to produce ALG and are readily available. Human thymocytes are used to produce ATG but are less readily available.

Polyclonal immunoglobulins form a heterogeneous group of antibodies, only a minority being specific to T-cells. They exert their effect by:
- complement mediated lysis of lymphocytes;
- clearance of lymphocytes by reticuloendothelial uptake;
- increasing the suppressor cell population;
- masking T-cell antigens.

The net result is a prompt and profound lymphopenia. Apart from treatment of severe rejection, polyclonal IgG has been used prior to grafting. Treatment is usually for 10–14 days.

Side effects

Overimmunosuppression with resultant infective or malignant complications is a concern. Repeat usage is limited by antibody formation. Immediate problems include chills, fever, rash and anaphylactic shock. There is wide batch to batch variation, and so the dose also varies by product and even by batch.

Monoclonal antibodies

These were developed against the T-cell. The commercially available preparation is OKT3, and is mainly used in reversal of severe rejection. As with ATG, OKT3 has been used prophylactically in high risk groups, such as in those who have rejected a previous graft.
- OKT3 does not remove all T-cells, but blocks T-cells which become

'blinded' to the antigens of the allograft, halting rejection. It binds to the CD3 protein at an antigenic site.

- It blocks cytotoxic T-lymphocyte mediated cell lysis and other T-cell functions. Mode of action is similar to polyclonals but is possibly more specific.
- In cadaveric grafts with acute rejection, 94% were reversed by OKT3 compared to 75% with high dose pulse steroid therapy, which was also translated into better graft survival at 1 year.

Side effects and treatment
Therapy is given with patients being monitored in hospital. Patients who are fluid overloaded should not receive OKT3 until they have had this corrected. This is due to the risk of pulmonary oedema as a result of capillary leak syndrome. Most patients develop a flu-like syndrome with fever, chills, nausea, diarrhoea, headache, etc. These symptoms can be reduced by prior administration of steroids and antihistamines. The dose for severe rejection is 5 mg/day for 5–14 days and its effect can be monitored by measuring the absolute T-lymphocyte count.

Therapeutic strategies

Cyclosporin monotherapy
CsA alone at 15–17.5 mg/kg/day given in two divided doses to maintain trough levels at 200–300 ng/ml. This strategy is not commonly used. Only a restricted number of transplant centres use this regime and only then for well matched donor/recipient combinations.

Combination therapy
Schedule 1: Cyclosporin dual therapy. Induction with CsA 10–15 mg/kg/day in two divided doses with Pred at 20–30 mg/day. Dose reduction: initially trough CsA levels are maintained higher at 200–300 ng/ml but this is reduced around three months to 100–200 ng/ml. Pred is also reduced in a step wise manner.

Schedule 2: Azathioprine dual therapy. This regime was used prior to the advent of CsA and is less effective in reducing acute rejection. Aza is given at 2.5 mg/kg/day as a single dose with Pred 20–30 mg/day (0.2–0.5 mg/kg/day depending on high or low dose philosophy). The two drugs are reduced with time as the renal function stabilizes (Aza 1–1.5 mg/kg/day together with steroid reduction).

Schedule 3: Cyclosporin triple therapy. This is now the commonest combination used. Acute rejection is reduced and CsA toxicity is minimized due to lower dosages being required. CsA dosage initially 5–12.5 mg/ kg/day, Aza 1–1.5 mg/kg/day and Pred 20–30 mg/day. Dosages of CsA are reduced with time lowering the trough level towards 100 ng/ ml. Pred is also withdrawn, the preferred long-term maintenance being CsA/Aza dual therapy if possible.

Schedule 4: Quadruple therapy. This strategy is used for the highest risk renal transplant and for pancreatic transplantation. Induction OKT3 or ATG is followed by CsA based triple therapy. The risk of rejection is highest during the first 3 months and the higher doses are given during this period. Dose reduction is usual after this. This combination has a 20% risk of acute rejection. Maintenance doses are continued indefinitely. This regime is now being replaced by triple therapy with the newer agents of FK 506 (tacrolimus), mycophenolate mofetil (MMF) in combination with Pred. This approach is favoured now as it reduces the risk of lymphoma which is not infrequently seen with the use of polyclonal and monoclonal antibodies.

Further reading

Morris PJ, Chan L, French ME, Ting A (1982). Low dose oral prednisolone in renal transplantation. *Lancet*, **1**, 525–527.

Kahan BD (1993). Optimization of Cyclosporine therapy. *Transplant Proc*, **25** (Suppl. 3), 5–9.

Wadhwa NK, Schroeder TJ, Pesce AJ *et al.* (1987). Cyclosporine drug interactions: a review. *Ther Drug Monit*, **9**, 399–406.

Myers BD (1989). What is Cyclosporine nephrotoxicity? *Tranpslant Proc*, **21**, 1430–1432.

Kahan BD (1985). Clinical summation. An algorithm for the management of patients with Cyclosporine-induced renal dysfunction. *Transplant Proc*, **17** (Suppl. 1), 303–308.

Goldstein G (1987). Overview of the development of Orthoclone OKT3: monoclonal antibody for therapeutic use in transplantation. *Transplant Proc*, **19** (Suppl. 1), 1–6.

Andreu J, Campistol JM, Oppenheimer F *et al.* (1994). Cyclosporine monotherapy as primary immunosuppression in renal transplantation: five-year experience. *Transplant Proc*, **26**, 337–340.

Loertscher R, Blier L, Steinmetz O, Nohr C (1992). The utility of Cyclosporine weaning in renal transplantation. *Ann Surg*, **215**, 368–376.

Allograft Dysfunction

Definition

Allograft dysfunction is defined as a rising serum creatinine with or without oliguria, proteinuria and metabolic derangements.

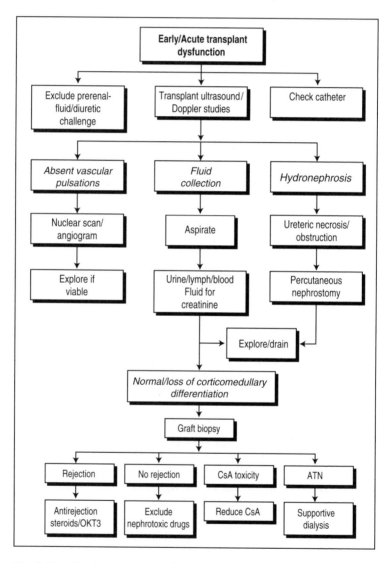

Fig. 2 Algorithm for management of acute renal transplant dysfunction.

Primary non-function

Intraoperative blue kidney
- Hyperacute rejection: usually after initial establishment of perfusion the kidney turns dusky, dark blue and soft. Urine production which may have been present stops. This is due to preformed antibodies or ABO incompatibility and requires graft removal.
- Arterial thrombosis/compression: kidney is usually soft and arterial pulsations are weak or absent. Does not have the dark colour of hyperacute rejection. Revision of anastomosis is indicated.
- Venous thrombosis/compression: initially well perfused kidney turns turgid with the capsule beginning to tear. Arterial pulsations still present. No flow present in the vein. Revise anastomosis.
- Acute Cyclosporin nephrotoxicity after rapid intravenous administration.

Acute tubular necrosis
By far the commonest cause with cadaveric kidneys is acute tubular necrosis (ATN) (44%) and is related to donor hypotension and prolonged warm and cold ischaemia times. Ischaemic ATN may be aggravated by CsA toxicity. Strategies to reduce this include intraoperative hydration, mannitol, avoidance of initial CsA, use of drugs to prevent reperfusion injury and special perfusion fluids. The incidence in live donors is exceedingly low.

Early/acute dysfunction (Fig. 2)
After initial establishment of renal function, the cause of dysfunction may be as follows.

Prerenal
- hypovolaemia
- hypotension
- congestive failure.

Postrenal
- obstruction of catheter/ureter
- sloughed/necrotic ureter
- extrinsic compression by blood, urinoma, lymphocoele
- ureteric stenosis.

Renal
1 Rejection

accelerated
acute vascular
acute cellular.
2 Drug
CsA
CsA interactions
drug induced interstitial nephritis
direct, e.g. aminoglycoside.
3 Infection
pyelonephritis
cytomegalovirus glomerulonephropathy.
4 Recurrent/*de novo* glomerular disease
5 Acute tubular necrosis
6 Vascular compromise

Late dysfunction

This is usually seen around 3 months after transplantation:
- transplant renal artery stenosis
- ureteric stenosis
- acute/chronic rejection
- recurrent/*de novo* glomerular disease
- chronic dysfunction due to hyperfiltration injury
- hypertension.

In the latter group when no treatable cause is found, aggressive management of hypertension with drugs, and if necessary with native kidney nephrectomy combined with dietary protein restriction, has been shown to slow the decline, which nevertheless is inevitable.

Further reading

Iwaki Y, Terasaki PI (1987). Primary nonfunction in human cadaver kidney transplantation: evidence for hidden hyperacute rejection. *Clin Transplant*, **1**, 125–127.

Parrott NR (1995). Early graft loss: the Cinderella of transplantation. *Nephrol Dial Transplant*, **10** (Suppl. 1), 32–35.

Urological Aspects

Ureteric

The ureter is the most common cause of postoperative complications.

This is usually due to technical reasons as is borne out by the wide variation in the reported incidence of complications from different centres.

Blood supply
The upper ureteric blood supply is usually from a ureteric branch of the lower polar or segmental artery. Preservation of this branch during donor nephrectomy is achieved by avoiding entry into the tissues in the triangle between the hilum, the gonadal vein and the upper ureter. Preservation of the perinephric fat ensures this. Preservation of all small lower polar branches is also important.

How long should the ureter be?
Initially long ureters were used. The minimum length to achieve a straight ureter after a no-tension ureteric anastomosis is ideal. The vascular anastomosis, therefore, should be as low as possible on the iliacs. A short ureter is less prone to kinking and ischaemic necrosis.

Where and how to implant
The anterior extravesical implant has the least morbidity.
- A lateral implantation site is preferable to the dome.
- The dome is mobile and may cause some degree of obstruction as the bladder fills up.
- Caliectasia in such transplants has been shown to regress as the bladder empties.
- The site should not be close to the bladder neck or too anterior as it is useful to have endoscopic access in case of late complications.
- A tunnelled implant avoiding reflux is advantageous.

While there has been no difference in the incidence of urinary infection with refluxing ureters, there has been a reported increased incidence of proteinuria, microhaematuria, hypertension and graft failure.

Urinary leak
Acute obstruction or leakage can occur due to ureteric necrosis. This is due to:
- ischaemia
- rejection
- infarction
- infection.

Anastomotic or vesical leakage is also possible, especially after the Leadbetter–Politano implant. This is manifested by:
- increased output from a drain

- rising creatinine
- expanding perigraft collection
- unexplained fever
- scrotal, labial or ipsilateral thigh swelling.

Diagnosis is confirmed by ultrasonography, measurement of the creatinine level in the drainage fluid or by isotope scintigraphy, the late images of which will show increased activity around the graft, after bladder emptying.

Small vesical leaks can be managed by bladder drainage for a further period. Ureteric leaks are best treated at once and may be managed in several ways.

- Percutaneously if small and amenable to such manoeuvres.
- By surgical re-exploration and a fresh reimplant if there is sufficient neoureter.
- By using the native ureter to perform a ureteroureterostomy or ureteropyelostomy over a stent.
- In cases of poor vascularity it may be possible to support the suture line using a pedicle of omentum.

Ureteric stenosis

Late ureteric stenosis occurs secondary to fibrosis or chronic ischaemia. It presents as progressive hydronephrosis and uraemia. Confirmation is by ultrasound scanning, nuclear studies or by percutaneous nephrostogram. Long tortuous ureters may be more susceptible. Management is by percutaneous or endoscopic balloon dilatation, or by surgery as for urine leak.

Lymphocoele

Lymphocoeles are usually seen in the immediate post-transplant period. There is anecdotal evidence that they may be more common after rejection.

- Differentiation from a urinoma is achieved by comparing the creatinine of the fluid aspirated with that of urine and serum— lymphatic creatinine is identical to that of serum.
- Lymph collections are usually amenable to percutaneous drainage.
- If they recur repeatedly they need surgical marsupialization by creating a peritoneal window.

Calyceal fistula

There have been instances of segmental parenchymal infarction after thrombosis or ligation of polar arterial branches. However, this is not common and may be related to larger branches being damaged. Lower polar branches need to be preserved to prevent ureteric necrosis.

Neoplasia
The incidence of neoplasia in renal allograft recipients is 100 times that of the general population. Neoplasia often appears after many months of immunosuppression (average 29 months).
- Epithelial tumours (40%) predominate followed by lympho-proliferative malignancies (20%).
- Cutaneous malignancy is the most common malignancy, with squamous cell carcinoma predominating over basal cell carcinoma.
- Non-Hodgkin's lymphomas are next in incidence followed by carcinoma of the cervix and uterus.
- Kaposi's sarcoma (300–400 times higher risk), carcinoma of the perineum or vulva, leukaemia and soft tissue sarcomas are more common than in the general population.

Lymphoma is often extranodal and the brain is the sole organ affected; it should be considered in the diagnosis of any central nervous system abnormality. Mortality from lymphoma is also much higher than that in the general population.
- Alterations in the immune surveillance system may allow malignancies to become established.
- Chronic stimulation of the reticuloendothelial system may be the cause of lymphoid malignancies.
- Latent oncogenic viruses may be activated in immunosuppressed hosts, there being an association between papillomavirus and the development of squamous skin cancer, cervical carcinoma and condylomata acuminata.
- *de novo* malignancy can be transmitted from the donor by the allograft.

Therapy
- Standard treatment as for each malignancy.
- Reduction or cessation of immunosuppression has been effective for Kaposi's sarcoma and lymphomas.
- Aza is discontinued during chemotherapy due to the risk of additive myelosuppression.
- Prompt removal of the allograft for *de novo* malignancy.
- Preventive care should include looking for dermatological and pelvic malignancies, and to biopsy any atypical lesion.

Further reading

Salvatierra O, Jr, Olcott C, Amend WJ, Jr, Cochrum KC, Feduska NJ (1977). Urological complications of renal transplantation can be prevented or controlled. *J Urol*, **117**, 421–424.

Benoit G, Blanchet P, Moukarzel M *et al.* (1994). Surgical complications in kidney transplantation. *Transplant Proc*, **26**, 287–288.

Thrasher JB, Temple DR, Spees EK (1990). Extravesical versus Leadbetter–Politano ureteroneocystostomy: a comparison of urological complications in 320 renal transplants. *J Urol*, **144**, 1105–1109.

Mathew TH, Kincaid-Smith P, Vikraman P (1977). Risks of vesicoureteric reflux in the transplanted kidney. *N Engl J Med*, **297**, 414–418.

Shah S, Nath V, Gopalkrishnan G, Pandey AP, Shastri JCM (1988). Evaluation of extravesical and Leadbetter–Politano ureteroneocystostomy in renal transplantation. *Br J Urol*, **62**, 412–413.

Loughlin KR, Tilney NL, Richie JP (1984). Urological complications in 718 renal transplant patients. *Surgery*, **95**, 297–302.

Penn I (1988). Transmission of cancer with organ donors. *Transplant Proc*, **20**, 739–740.

Penn I (1983). Renal transplantation in patients with pre-existing malignancies. *Transplant Proc*, **15**, 1079–1081.

Oncology I

Partial Nephrectomy for Renal Cell Carcinoma

Introduction

Renal sparing surgery dates from the late 1800s but fell into disfavour due to early problems with renal bleeding, urinary fistulae and a high postoperative mortality. In 1950 Vermooten advocated conservative surgery for renal cell carcinoma (RCC) based on his observation that these tumours formed a pseudocapsule, but its popularity again waned after Robson's demonstration in 1969 of improved survival after extrafascial nephrectomy. However, with increasing detection of incidental low-stage RCC there is renewed enthusiasm for this form of surgery, which now appears to give satisfactory long-term survival, principally due to improved patient selection, recent advances in renal imaging and renal vascular surgery for other conditions, as well as improved methods of preventing ischaemia.

The role of partial nephrectomy for unilateral RCC (including the unsuspected RCC) with a normal contralateral kidney remains controversial. There are several strong arguments in favour of radical surgery under such circumstances, perhaps the most persuasive being a local recurrence rate of 7–10% following partial nephrectomy compared to 1–2% after radical nephrectomy and additionally unsuspected multifocal tumour in a proportion of cases. Currently, the EORTC (study 30904) is conducting a multicentre clinical trial to address this question.

Indications for partial nephrectomy
- Bilateral synchronous RCC.
- RCC in an anatomically/functionally solitary kidney.
- Unilateral RCC in patients with a functioning contralateral kidney, and any concomitant condition with the potential for adversely affecting future renal function (e.g. calculi or renal artery disease).
- Unilateral RCC in patients with a functioning but impaired contralateral kidney (renal artery stenosis, hydronephrosis, chronic pyelonephritis, reflux, systemic disease, e.g. diabetes, nephrocalcinosis).
- RCC in von Hippel–Lindau disease.

Additional preoperative evaluation
- Selective renal angiography.

- Good preoperative hydration.
- Patients <60 years with bilateral RCC—screen blood DNA to exclude Von Hippel–Lindau disease (VHL).

Surgical technique
(as described by AC Novick of the Cleveland Clinic where by December 1994, 327 patients had undergone renal sparing surgery for sporadic RCC).
- Incision through the bed of 11/12th rib.
- Mobilization of the kidney and perinephric fat, leaving fat over tumour.
- Regional hypothermia and renal artery occlusion in most cases (except small polar tumours)—gives 3 hours protection from ischaemia.
- Kidney is placed in a bowel bag.
- Immediately prior to renal artery occlusion, 12.5g of intravenous (IV) mannitol given.
- Renal artery clamped and kidney immediately covered in sterile ice slush.
- Kidney left for 15 minutes to allow core temperature to drop to 20°C.
- Renal vein left unclamped allowing retrograde renal oxygenation.
- Anticoagulation not routinely used.
- Wedge excision used for most tumours on renal surface.
- One to 2 cm of normal kidney should be excised, and frozen section (or possibly intraoperative ultrasound scan (USS)) should be performed to ensure tumour free margins.
- Haemostasis using suture ligation or argon beam coagulator.
- Openings into the collecting system closed with absorbable suture.
- Renal parenchyma reapproximated over a haemostatic plug.
- Renal artery clamp removed and haemostasis secured.

Technique of excision
(depends on size and location of tumour)
- Wedge excision.
- Polar segmental nephrectomy.
- Major transverse resection (ureteric stent may be needed following this).
- Extracorporeal partial nephrectomy/autotransplantation (large central tumours).
- Enucleation is problematic and should be reserved for cases of von Hippel–Lindau disease in which multiple RCCs are often located within cysts.

Bilateral RCC
- Staged bilateral partial nephrectomies.
- Partial nephrectomy and radical nephrectomy, with the less involved side done first—obviates the need for temporary dialysis if partial nephrectomy is complicated by postoperative acute tubular necrosis (ATN).
- A renal remnant of at least 20% of one normal kidney is necessary to remain dialysis-independent.

Predisposing factors for acute renal failure
- solitary kidney
- tumour > 7 cm
- >50% parenchymal excision
- >60 minutes ischaemia time
- *ex vivo* surgery.

Late sequelae
- proteinuria, treated by low protein diet and ACE inhibitors
- glomerulosclerosis
- progressive renal failure.

Recommended follow-up (See Hafez *et al.*, 1997)
- T1: no invasive monitoring needed.
- T2: annual CXR, abdominal CT every 2 years.
- T3: same as T2 except should have CT every 6 months during first 2 years of follow-up.

Outcome of surgery
Radical nephrectomy versus conservative surgery for stage T1 or T2 renal cell carcinoma (Table 5).

Table 5 Outcome of radical surgery versus conservative surgery in T1/T2 renal carcinoma.

	5 year survival (%)	
Reference	Radical surgery	Conservative surgery
Robson *et al.* (*J Urol*, 101, 1969)	66	—
Skinner *et al.* (*Cancer*, 28, 1971)	68	—
Lieber *et al.* (*J Urol*, 125, 1981)	79	—
Novick *et al.* (*J Urol*, 141, 1989)	—	90
Morgan & Zincke (*J Urol*, 144, 1990)	—	90
Butler *et al.* (*Urology*, 45, 1995)	97	100

Based on these figures, some have recommended expanding the indications for conservative renal surgery to include those patients with small (<4 cm), low-stage, peripherally located tumours and a normal contralateral kidney.

Further reading
Novick AC, Streem S, Montie JE *et al.* (1989). Conservative surgery for renal cell carcinoma: a single centre experience with 100 patients. *J Urol,* **141**, 835–839.

Klein EA, Novick AC (1992). Partial nephrectomy for renal cell carcinoma. In: *Advances in Urology,* Vol. 5 (eds B Lytton, WJ Catalona, LI Lipshultz, EJ McGuire), pp. 1–9. Mosby Year Book, St Louis.

Thrasher JB, Robertson JE, Paulson DF (1994). Expanding indications for conservative renal surgery in renal cell carcinoma. *Urology,* **43**, 160–168.

Campbell SC, Novick AC, Streem SB, Klein E, Licht M (1994). Complications of nephron sparing surgery for renal tumours. *J Urol,* **151**, 1177–1180.

Hafez KS, Novick AC, Campbell SC (1997). Patterns of tumour recurrence and guidelines for follow-up after nephron sparing surgery for sporadic renal cell carcinoma. *J Urol,* **157**, 2067–2070.

Von Hippel–Lindau Disease

Introduction
- Von Hippel–Lindau disease (VHL) is rare (1 in 36 000 live births).
- Autosomal dominant trait.
- Predisposition to develop retinal angiomas (60%), haemangioblastomas of the brain and spinal cord (60%), RCC (45%), phaeochromocytomas (18%), cystadenomas of the pancreas and epididymis, and islet cell carcinomas of the pancreas.
- Individuals who inherit the disease gene may remain free of such manifestations or may develop tumours in one or more systems.

VHL and RCC
- RCC occurs in approximately 45% of patients with VHL.
- Histologically clear cell.
- Often multifocal, bilateral.
- Mean age at diagnosis is 39 years.
- Thirty to 35% risk of tumour progression and death.

VHL gene
- Cloned in 1993.
- Located to a segment between *RAF*-1 oncogene (chromosome 3p25) and D3S18, a polymorphic DNA marker at 3p26.

- Belongs to a family of tumour-suppressor genes.
- Specific types of mutation correlate with specific phenotypic expression.
- Probe 64E2 is a distal flanking marker.
- Contains three exons.
- Encodes a 284 amino acid protein.

Screening and molecular genetics

- Early diagnosis might prevent death from haemangioblastomas (using MRI) and RCCs (using CT).
- Until recently the only approach to early diagnosis was periodic examination of the eye, brain and abdomen in all asymptomatic members of VHL families.
- Prior to cloning the VHL gene, the identification of probes that flank the disease gene meant it was possible to identify carriers of the disease gene by DNA polymorphism analysis. Linehan and coworkers at the National Cancer Institute (NCI) collected blood from 182 members of 16 families with VHL. Forty-eight asymptomatic, at risk individuals were examined for occult disease and also tested by DNA polymorphism analysis. DNA polymorphisms predicted nine gene carriers (all had evidence of occult disease), 33 had a normal gene (32 no evidence of occult disease) and in six cases the test was not informative.
- DNA-based diagnostic-testing is now available to allow determination of carrier status.

Natural history

- In order to determine the natural history of the renal lesions in VHL, a serial CT study has been performed on 28 patients.
- Patients were followed for a mean of 2.4 years (range 1–12 years).
- The 28 patients had 228 renal lesions (average eight per patient).
- On CT appearance, 168 (74%) were classified as cysts, 18 (8%) as cysts with solid components and 42 (18%) as solid masses.
- Among 12 patients with pathologic confirmation, the solid components of cysts and the solid lesions almost always contained RCC.
- The majority of cysts remained the same size (71%) or enlarged (20%); 9% became smaller.
- Although it is generally thought that cysts are precursors of cancers, the transformation of a simple cyst to a solid lesion was observed in only two patients.
- The great majority (40/42) solid lesions enlarged (doubling time = 10 months).
- These authors recommend surgery be performed when the renal tumours approach 3 cm in size, based on the fact that until this size is reached the chances of metastases are low.

- In patients with multiple fast growing tumours one should consider bilateral nephrectomy followed immediately by renal transplantation.

Surgical management
The results of nephron sparing surgery for VHL are less satisfactory than for sporadic RCC. In essence, the risk of tumour progression and death following partial nephrectomy in these patients is unidentified and these patients have a high risk of local tumour recurrence. Consequently, it is not known whether renal tumours in VHL are best managed by partial nephrectomy to preserve renal function or by immediate bilateral nephrectomy with subsequent renal replacement therapy.

- A multicentre report of surgery in 65 patients with VHL was recently reported (Steinbach *et al.*, *J Urol* 1995).
- Fifty-four patients had bilateral and 11 unilateral surgery.
- Sixteen had radical and 49 partial nephrectomy.
- Of the latter, 51% developed recurrent tumour but only two patients developed metastases at a mean follow-up of 68 months.
- Five and 10 year survival rates for the group undergoing partial nephrectomy were 100% and 81%.
- End-stage renal failure occurred in 23% of patients.

Further reading
Glenn GM, Linehan WM, Hosoe S *et al.* (1992). Screening for von Hippel–Lindau disease by DNA polymorphism analysis. *JAMA*, **267**, 1226–1231.

Choyke PL, Glenn GM, Walther MM *et al.* (1992). The natural history of renal lesions in von Hippel–Lindau disease: a serial CT study in 28 patients. *AJR*, **159**, 1229–1234.

Novick AC, Streem SB (1992). Long-term follow up after nephron sparing surgery for renal cell carcinoma in von Hippel–Lindau disease. *J Urol*, **147**, 1488–1490.

Steinbach F, Novick AC, Zincke H *et al.* (1995). Treatment of renal cell carcinoma in von Hippel–Lindau disease: a multicenter study. *J Urol*, **153**, 1812–1816.

Carcinoma *in situ* of the Penis

Nomenclature and incidence
- The terms carcinoma *in situ* (CIS) of the penis, erythroplasia of Queyrat and Bowen's disease are interchangeable.
- The incidence of CIS penis is likely to increase with the increased prevalence of human papillomavirus (HPV) infection.
- The natural history of CIS penis is that approximately 10% of men will later develop invasive penile carcinoma.

Bowen's disease
- Squamous cell carcinoma of the skin *in situ* was described by Bowen in 1912 in two patients with non-genital lesions.
- Bowen's disease of the penis is usually an erythematous plaque on the glans which is round or slightly irregular, usually 1–1.5 cm in diameter.
- There are reports that Bowen's disease is associated with visceral tumours but several studies do not support this.

Erythroplasia of Queyrat
- Originally described by Queyrat in 1911.
- The definitive study of erythroplasia of Queyrat was reported by Graham and Helwig in *Cancer* in 1973. In this study of 100 cases, approximately 50% of lesions were single and 50% were multifocal. Of 87 patients in whom the information was available 84 (95%) were uncircumcised. Lesions were described as shiny, erythematous, velvety plaques that were slightly raised. The initial complaint was of redness, crusting and scaling and more than 50% noted itching and/ or pain.

CIS penis and HPV
Infection with HPV may be an important factor in the development of CIS penis. Recent studies, using polymerase chain reaction (PCR) based techniques, suggest HPV type 16 DNA can be detected in approximately 50% of cases of invasive squamous cell carcinoma (SCC) of the penis but in a much higher proportion of cases (>90%) of CIS penis.

Histological features of CIS
- Parakeratosis.
- Hyperkeratosis.
- Papillomatosis.
- Thinning of the granular layer.
- Acanthosis.
- Elongation and broadening of the rete ridges.
- Atypia of the keratinocytes.
- Pleomorphic nuclear hyperchromaticity.
- Mitotic activity in all layers of the epidermis.
- Chronic inflammatory infiltrate in the underlying dermis.

Differential diagnosis
- invasive SCC

- balanitis circinata (associated with Reiter's syndrome)
- candidal balanitis
- Zoon's balanitis (balanitis circumscripta plasma cellularis—a rare disorder that tends to occur in elderly uncircumcised men)
- penile psoriasis
- fixed drug eruptions.

Accurate diagnosis depends on biopsy. Small lesions can be totally excised, larger lesions require punch biopsy to a depth of 3–5 mm.

Treatment
- Circumcision is generally recommended.
- Laser surgery: The CO_2 or Nd:YAG lasers have a role after histological confirmation of the diagnosis and after invasive SCC has been excluded. The CO_2 laser has a wavelength of 10 600 nm and primarily carbonizes/vaporizes tissues with minimal tissue penetration into deeper layers. The procedure can be performed using local anaesthesia. The lesion plus a margin of 5 mm of surrounding epithelium should be destroyed to a depth of 2.5 mm. It is possible to completely remove the epithelium from the glans and inner prepuce with satisfactory cosmetic and functional results. The Nd:YAG laser causes protein denaturation and emits a wavelength of 1060 nm—tissue penetration of several millimetres is achieved.
- Surgical excision with adequate margins (5 mm). It is essential to remove deeper layers to assess for invasive malignancy.
- Alternative surgical approaches include micrographic surgery (Mohs, 1985).
- Local radiotherapy has been used but data regarding its use are limited.
- Others have used topical 5-fluorouracil with good results in small numbers of patients.

Bowenoid papulosis
- Originally described in 1977.
- Lesions appear as rounded, reddish to violaceous papules arising on the glans or more commonly on the shaft of the penis.
- In contrast to CIS penis, the typical patient at diagnosis is significantly younger (20–35 years), circumcised and is often sexually promiscuous.
- This lesion is also associated with HPV.
- Histologically it is very similar to CIS penis but the latter has a significantly greater degree of atypia which should allow distinction.

- Despite the similar histology, Bowenoid papulosis is completely benign although is associated with cervical carcinoma in sexual partners.
- Standard treatment is superficial excision although the other modalities listed above have all been used.

Further reading

Gerber GS (1994). Carcinoma *in situ* of the penis. *J Urol*, **151**, 829–833.

Cupp MR, Malek RS, Goellner JR, Smith TF, Espy MJ (1995). The detection of human papillomavirus deoxyribonucleic acid in intraepithelial, *in situ*, verrucous and invasive carcinoma of the penis. *J Urol*, **154**, 1024–1029.

Graham JH, Helwig EB (1973). Erythroplasia of Queyrat. A clinicopathologic and histochemical study. *Cancer*, **32**, 1396–1414.

Mohs FE, Snow SN, Messing EM *et al.* (1985). Microscopically controlled surgery in the treatment of carcinoma of the penis. *J Urol*, **133**, 961–966.

Viral Agents and Carcinoma of the Penis

Introduction

- Squamous cell carcinoma of the penis (SCCP) is uncommon and accounts for less than 1% of adult male cancers in developed countries.
- The combination of multiple carcinogenic factors coupled with the current rapid rise in immunologic disorders is likely to lead to a substantial increase in the historically low incidence of SCCP, particularly in the USA.
- SCCP usually occurs in elderly uncircumcised males in whom there is a significant correlation with poor hygiene.
- There are two direct lines of evidence that suggest a viral role in the aetiology of SCCP. There is, first, epidemiological and, second, *in vitro* evidence of the transforming potential of viruses with known trophisms for genital tissues, in particular human papillomavirus (HPV) and herpes simplex type-2 (HSV-2).
- The same viruses are implicated in the pathogenesis of cervical cancer but there are distinct differences in that cervical cancer accounts for 4500 cases per annum in England and Wales, compared with 300 cases of penile cancer, and cervical cancer occurs from the third decade onwards unlike carcinoma of the penis. It is clear, therefore, that factors other than a sexually transmissible tumorigenic virus must also be important.

Links with carcinoma of the cervix

- There is an increased risk of cervical cancer in the partners of men with penile cancer, suggesting a transmissible cofactor.
- A major component of the evidence that viruses may be aetiologically important in cervical cancer lies in the detection of particular HPV subtypes (16 and 18 in the UK) in association with cervical cancers and CIN, and a lack of association with other subtypes (6 and 11 in the UK) known to cause benign lesions.
- Studies in male sexual partners of women with carcinoma of the cervix reveal a high incidence of asymptomatic lesions detectable by cytological/brush techniques in which HPV DNA (6, 11, 16 and 18) can be detected.

Acetoacid whitening

- Acetoacid has been used to identify HPV infection of grossly normal cervical tissue in women undergoing colposcopy. The opacity displayed reflects hypercellularity and protein coagulation.
- In men, 5% acetic acid-soaked gauze is applied to the penis and left for 5–15 minutes.
- When acetoacid whitening is present, biopsy is mandatory to confirm the histopathologic presence of HPV infection.

Studies of HPV

- Early studies to detect HPV in penile cancers were unsuccessful, probably because of insufficient sensitivity of the methods used.
- The advent of methods employing the PCR has changed this and in the past few years at least three good studies examining HPV in SCCP/CIS penis have been reported. Malek studied 34 men with precancerous and cancerous squamous cell lesions of the penis and from 20 representative patients using PCR amplification detected HPV DNA in 80%. Weiner performed a retrospective analysis of a 20 year experience in a single institution in which he reported HPV DNA in 9/29 (31%) patients with invasive SCCP (HPV 16 DNA in 8 and HPV 18 DNA in 1). Of patients with CIS penis, one of two was positive for HPV type 16. Sarkar has performed the biggest study of CIS penis (15 cases—seven Bowenoid and eight non-Bowenoid, as well as 11 cases of invasive SCCP). All seven of the Bowenoid forms of CIS penis were positive for HPV 16 DNA which was also detected in 9/11 cases of invasive SCCP.
- It is now emerging that the Bowenoid forms of intraepithelial neoplasia and most SCCPs contain the E6 to E7 portion of type 16 HPV.

Further reading

Malek RS, Goellner JR, Smith TF, Espy MJ, Cupp MR (1993). Human papillomavirus infection and intraepithelial, *in situ*, and invasive carcinoma of the penis. *Urology*, **42**, 159–170.

Weiner JS, Effert PJ, Humphrey PA, Yu L, Liu ET, Walter PJ (1992). Prevalence of human papillomavirus types 16 and 18 in squamous-cell carcinoma of the penis: a retrospective analysis of primary and metastatic lesions by differential polymerase chain reaction. *Int J Cancer*, **50**, 694–701.

Sarkar FH, Miles BJ, Plieth DH, Crissman JD (1992). Detection of human papillomavirus in squamous neoplasm of the penis. *J Urol*, **147**, 389–392.

James N, Crook T (1992). Viruses and penile cancer. In: *Urological Oncology* (eds J Waxman, G Williams), pp. 43–47. Edward Arnold, London.

Carcinoma *in situ* of the Testis

Introduction

- The contralateral testes of men with testicular cancer, testes from infertile men and those with a history of maldescent may contain premalignant cells— CIS (intratubular germ cell neoplasia, ITGN).
- Skakkebaek (Danish andrologist) was the first to describe CIS testis in a report in the *Lancet* in 1972.
- Skakkebaek's group subsequently reported detection of CIS of the contralateral testis in 27/500 (5.4%) cases of unilateral testicular germ cell cancer (see Von der Maase, *BMJ*, 1986).
- The incidence of CIS in the contralateral testis has been confirmed by a German study of 1954 men with unilateral testis cancer who had a contralateral testis biopsy. CIS testis was detected in 4.9% of men and although a history of undescent/testicular atrophy increased the risk, 64% of cases occurred in normal testes.
- CIS testis is most commonly seen in seminiferous tubules adjacent to a germ cell tumour.
- Occurs in 2% of biopsy specimens from men with a history of cryptorchidism.
- Occurs in 0.4–1% of specimens from infertile men.
- Risk may be as high as 80% in men who have gonadal dysgenesis, androgen insensitivity or a 45XO, 46XY karyotype.
- CIS testis appears to have the potential to progress to both semino-matous and non-seminomatous germ cell tumours and the risk is substantial (50% at 5 years).
- Bilateral testis cancer is reported to occur in 1–2% of men, but this figure seems to be rising, perhaps due to improved survival rates

resulting in a larger population at risk. Most bilateral cancers are diagnosed sequentially.

Detection
- Testicular biopsy is the only reliable method of detecting CIS testis although the abnormal cells may be missed by this technique.
- Abnormal cells seem to spread throughout the testis and are therefore likely to be detected by random biopsy. Experimental studies have shown that a 3–4mm biopsy will be positive if only 5% of the tubules are involved with CIS testis. To support this, none of the 473 men with a negative biopsy from Skakkebaek's series went on to develop invasive cancer.
- It is now standard practice in Denmark to carry out routine contra-lateral testicular biopsy although this policy has not been adopted elsewhere, particularly the USA where USS is used to subsequently monitor the contralateral testis, or the UK.
- The specimen should be fixed in Bouin's solution which preserves excellent nuclear detail and allows later immunohistochemical analysis.
- CIS cells as well as seminoma cells stain positively with placental alkaline phosphatase (PLAP). Recently new monoclonal antibodies M2A, 43-9F and TRA-1-60 have been reported to detect testicular CIS cells. These cells also appear to have high expression of the c-kit proto-oncogene and frequently demonstrate immunoreactivity for p53. The Danish group have also reported detection of hyperdiploid cells in seminal fluid using *in situ* hybridization and a probe for chromosome 1.

Histological features
- Malignant cells in a single row along the tubular membrane.
- Nuclei are enlarged and irregular with prominent and multiple nucleoli.
- Diameter of seminiferous tubules is reduced with only testicular CIS and Sertoli cells present.

Treatment
- Treatment depends on the status of the other testis.
- Unilateral CIS/normal contralateral testis—orchiectomy is recommended.
- With a clinically evident tumour and contralateral CIS testis a dose of 20 Gy of radiotherapy in 10 fractions is probably curative.
- The effectiveness of systemic chemotherapy, which will be indicated for a proportion of these patients is intriguing and controversial. It is

probable that the CIS testis cells are destroyed completely in some cases and incompletely in others. This situation is analogous to systemic chemotherapy for invasive bladder cancer and CIS bladder.

Further reading

Hargreave TB (1986). Carcinoma *in situ* of the testis. *Br Med J*, **293**, 1389–1390.

Von der Maase H, Rorth M, Walbom-Jorgensen S *et al.* (1986). Carcinoma *in situ* of contralateral testis in patients with testicular germ cell cancer: study of 27 cases in 500 patients. *Br Med J*, **293**, 1398–1401.

Montie JE (1993). Carcinoma *in situ* of the testis and bilateral carcinoma. *Urol Clin North Am*, **20**, 127–132.

Dieckman KP, Loy V (1996). Prevalence of contralateral testicular intraepithelial neoplasia in patients with testicular germ cell neoplasms. *J Clin Oncol*, **14**, 3126–3132.

Chemotherapy Regimens for Testis Cancer

Introduction

- The incidence of germ cell tumours of the testis is increasing (mainly in the age-group 15–19 years) in association with earlier onset of puberty and earlier onset of regular sexual intercourse.
- 1400 cases per annum in England and Wales.

Historical aspects

- Combination chemotherapy for testicular cancer was introduced by Li and Whitmore in 1960 and, although in these early days there was a good initial response rate, long-term survivors were uncommon.
- The current era of chemotherapy for germ cell tumours was heralded by the introduction (in the 1970s by Dr Einhorn at the University of Indiana) of high dose cisplatin into the combination of Vinblastine and Bleomycin (giving PVB) previously developed at the MD Anderson Hospital in Houston, Texas.
- The second milestone was the introduction of Etoposide (VP16), replacing Vinblastine, producing the BEP combination which has now become the 'gold standard' chemotherapy regimen.
- Approximately 75% of patients with metastatic teratoma present with low-volume, good prognosis disease and cure can be anticipated using BEP in at least 95% of these.

Indications for BEP
- Metastatic teratoma (Non-seminomatous germ cell tumour (NSGCT))—4 cycles of BEP.
- High risk (3 or 4 risk factors of vascular invasion, lymphatic invasion, the presence of undifferentiated cells, the absence of yolk sac elements); stage I NSGCT—2 cycles of BEP.
- Stage IIc, III and IV seminoma.

Standard regimen
Four cycles of BEP based on a 21 day cycle.
- Bleomycin (B): 30 U IV, days 2, 9, 16.
- Etoposide (E): 120 mg/m^2/day IV, days 1, 2, 3.
- Cisplatin (P): 20 mg/m^2/day IV, days 1, 2, 3, 4, 5.

Prognostic factors
The MRC have performed an analysis of prognostic factors in just under 800 patients with metastatic NSGCT treated between 1982 and 1988. From this, the adverse presentations of NSGCT are defined in Table 6 with the remaining patients forming the good prognosis group.

Table 6 NSGCT: definition of the adverse prognostic group

One of:
> 20 lung metastases
AFP > 1000 IU/l or hCG > 10 000 IU/l
Liver, bone or brain metastases
Mediastinal mass > 5 cm

With BEP alone, cure will be achieved in no more than 50% of poor prognosis patients. Currently at the Royal Marsden Hospital, poor risk NSGCT, as identified by MRC criteria, are treated with intensified chemotherapy using the C-BOP (Carboplatin, Bleomycin, Oncovin, Cisplatin)/BEP regimen. The MD Anderson schedule for poor risk groups alternates CISCA 2 (Adriamycin, Cyclophosphamide, Cisplatin) with VB-4 (Vinblastine and Bleomycin). An alternative effective multiple agent regimen is POMB-ACE (Cisplatin, Vincristine (Oncovin), Methotrexate, Bleomycin with Actinomycin-D, Cyclophosphamide and Etoposide) which was developed at Charing Cross Hospital in 1977. Recently the IGCCCG have defined prognostic categories (Table 7).

Table 7 International Germ Cell Cancer Collaborative Group: Prognostic categories.

	NSGCT		Seminoma	
Good prognosis	Testis/RP primary No non-pulmonary visceral mets AFP < 1000 ng/ml HCG < 5000 iu/L LDH < 1.5 × N	5 yr PFS 89% 5 yr survival 92%	Any primary site Any markers No non-pulmonary visceral mets	5 yr PFS 82% 5 yr survival 86%
Intermediate prognosis	Testis/RP primary No non-pulmonary visceral mets AFP : 1000–10 000 HCG : 5000–50 000 LDH : 1.5–10 × N	5 yr PFS 75% 5 yr survival 80%	Any primary site Any markers Non-pulmonary visceral mets	5 yr PFS 68% 5 yr survival 73%
Poor prognosis	Mediastinal primary Non-pulmonary visceral mets AFP > 10 000 HCG > 50 000 LDH > 10 × N	5 yr PFS 41% 5 yr survival 47%		

RP: retroperitoneal; PFS: progression free survival

Modified schedules

Several centres are currently attempting to modify these standard chemotherapy regimens in order to minimize drug toxicity. Although it has been conventional to use 4 cycles, the Indiana University group have reported identical results for good prognosis patients and a significant reduction in toxicity using only 3 cycles. There is a current EORTC/MRC (TE20) study comparing 3 with 4 cycles of BEP, in addition to comparing 3 with 5 days of treatment in good prognosis testis cancer.

Salvage chemotherapy

- Patients who fail standard platinum-based chemotherapy have a poor prognosis with survival of 20–30%.

- Vinblastine/Ifosphamide/Cisplatin will cure approximately 25% of patients when used as second line therapy.
- High-dose Carboplatin and Etoposide with autologous bone marrow transplantation can cure 15–20% of patients whose disease progressed during prior Cisplatin combination chemotherapy, or when the regimen is used as third line therapy or later chemotherapy.
- Paclitaxel has shown some effectiveness in treating patients with Cisplatin refractory disease, with a response rate of 26% overall in four consecutive series involving a total of 83 patients. The side effects of Paclitaxel include neutropenia, neurotoxicity and fatigue.
- Temezolamide demonstrates *in vitro* activity.

Chemotherapy for seminoma

Though testicular seminoma is almost as common as NSGCT it usually presents at an early stage not requiring chemotherapy. Furthermore, seminoma is exquisitely sensitive to radiotherapy, and therefore chemotherapy has not been extensively explored in early stages of the disease. Chemotherapy is, however, indicated for stage IIC (bulky para-aortic lymph nodes (PANs)), III and IV disease. Seminoma is highly sensitive to drug combinations containing Cisplatin. In general, the rarity of these tumours has led to their treatment with schedules developed for NSGCT, especially PVB and BEP. The results are excellent. The MRC is currently running a trial comparing single agent Carboplatin with more standard combinations of Etoposide and Cisplatin in patients with stage IIC, III and IV seminoma. An EORTC Study (30874) reports that Ifosphamide, Vincristine and Cisplatin together are highly effective in treating metastatic seminoma but comprise a highly toxic combination.

Further reading

Wilkins M, Horwich A (1996). Diagnosis and treatment of urological malignancy: the testes. *Br J Hosp Med*, **55**, 199–203.

Horwich A (1992). New cytotoxic chemotherapy programmes for advanced testicular cancer. In: *Urological Oncology* (eds J Waxman, G Williams), pp. 16–28. Edward Arnold, London.

Horwich A, Norman A, Fisher NC, Hendry WF, Nicholls J, Dearnaley DP (1994). Primary chemotherapy for Stage II nonseminomatous germ cell tumours of the testis. *J Urol*, **151**, 72–78.

Oncology II

Management of Localized Prostate Cancer

Introduction
- Approximately nine thousand deaths per year due to prostate cancer in England and Wales (1993).
- Approximately 60% of cases in the UK present with advanced disease.
- Majority of men are >70 years.
- Increasing numbers of TURPs in younger men and the increasing use of PSA testing will result in increased detection of localized disease.
- No randomized prospective study of accurately staged patients exists to compare the results of surgery with radiotherapy or watchful waiting in terms of survival.

Treatment options and guidelines
- Radical treatment is restricted to patients with stage T1 and T2 disease in whom metastatic disease has been excluded by bone scan.
- Patients opting for radical prostatectomy with PSA > 10 ng/ml or Gleason score > 7 will also require frozen sections of obturator nodes. All men should have a 10 year life expectancy or greater and be fully informed of the potential side effects of treatment.
- Radiotherapy is likely to be less effective in treating bulky disease and leads to higher local recurrence rates; this is offset by lesser risk of impotence and incontinence following radiotherapy.
- Ideally patients opting for treatment should take part in ongoing randomized studies.
- Patients opting for 'watchful waiting' require 3 monthly PSA measurement to monitor progression.

Progression
- Progression is related to cancer volume and tumour grade; the life expectancy of the patient may be more unpredictable.
- Johansson reported a disease specific mortality rate of 8.5% in 223 highly selected patients with localized prostate cancer followed up for 10 years. Forty-three per cent of patients demonstrated tumour progression but only 12% developed metastases.

- Lowe and Listrom (1988) reported 5 year progression rates in 232 T1 tumours—T1a:12%; T1b:53%.
- Data on T2 tumours are sparse and the picture is clouded by the recognized staging error between T2b, T2c and T3 disease. In a study of 56 T2 tumours, Adolfsson and Carstensen demonstrated: 49% local progression and 8% progression to metastases at 5 years; 72% local progression and 23% progression to metastases at 10 years.
- In a wide review of published data, Chodak reported 5 year progression rate (to metastasis) of 7% for G1 tumours, 16% for G2 tumours and 49% for G3 tumours (all stages).
- Clearly some tumours will progress without treatment and these are cases which will potentially benefit from radical treatment provided that the life expectancy of the patient is 10 years or greater.

Outcome
- In an attempt to assess quality of life as well as potential survival advantage from radical therapy, Fleming *et al.* (1993) used decision analysis to examine the impact of treatments on quality adjusted life expectancy for patients aged 60–75 years with localized prostate cancer. This study incorporated data from all published series of treated localized prostate cancer. Patients with well differentiated tumours did not obtain benefit in terms of quality adjusted life expectancy whereas those patients with moderately or poorly differentiated tumours did. The difference, however, was so small that 'watchful waiting' was felt to be a reasonable alternative. There is some criticism of the assumed progression rates in this paper.
- Catalona has recently reviewed the results of radical prostatectomy in 1000 patients treated at major North American centres. Five year actuarial (PSA-based) recurrence free survival post-radical prostatectomy (stage T1/T2): Baylor 92%, Duke 72%, Johns Hopkins 97%, UCLA 92%, Washington 91%. Catalona argues that anatomic radical retropubic prostatectomy provides 'unexcelled cancer control with low morbidity and until other treatments are proved as effective should be the preferred treatment for men with localized prostate cancer whose life expectancy exceeds 10 years'.
- One of the reservations concerning radical prostatectomy remains the positive margin rate, which is commonly as high as 30%.
- It is difficult to compare surgical series with series where patients have been treated using radical radiotherapy due to lack of pathological staging. A recent study (Powell) of 145 patients with

localized prostate cancer treated by radical radiotherapy after negative pelvic lymphadenectomy showed cancer specific survival at 10 and 15 years, of 84% and 80% respectively.

- Patient selection partially responsible for poor results from radiotherapy.
- Prostate intervention versus observation trial (PIVOT): study in the USA and Scandinavian study comparing radical prostatectomy with 'watchful waiting': data not available for 10 years.
- Randomized trials or a means of reliably predicting tumour behaviour provide the only means to reach rational decisions in the management of clinically localized prostate cancer.

Further reading

Adolfsson J, Carstensen J (1991). Natural course of clinically localised prostate adenocarcinoma in men less than 70 years old. *J Urol*, **146**, 96–98.

Catalona WJ (1995). Contemporary results with anatomic radical prostatectomy. *Cancer*, **75** (Suppl. 7), 1903–1908.

Chodak GW, Thisted RA, Gerber GS *et al.* (1994). Results of conservative management of clinically localised prostate cancer. *N Engl J Med*, **330**, 242–248.

Lowe BA, Listrom MB (1988). Incidental carcinoma of the prostate: an analysis of the predictors of progression. *J Urol*, **140**, 1340–1344.

Johansson JE, Adami HO, Andersson SO, Bergstrom R, Holberg L, Krusemo UB (1992). High 10 year survival rate in patients with early untreated prostate cancer. *JAMA*, **267**, 2191–2196.

Fleming C, Wasson JH, Albertsen PC, Barry MJ, Wennberg JE (1993). A decision analysis of alternative treatment strategies for clinically localised prostate cancer. *JAMA*, **269**, 2650–2658.

Powell CR, Huisman TK, Riffenburgh RH, Saunders EL, Bethel KJ, Johnstone PA (1997). Outcome for surgically staged localised prostate cancer treated with external beam radiation therapy. *J Urol*, **157**, 1754–1759.

Treatment of Metastatic Prostate Cancer

Total androgen blockade

Adrenal androgens, dihydroepiandrostenedione and androstenedione are converted peripherally to testosterone and dihydrotestosterone (DHT). They contribute up to 20% of the total dihydrotestosterone in the prostate. The rationale behind total androgen blockade is the hypothesis that androgens produced from the adrenal may cause tumour progression. Antiandrogens would block these androgens at the androgen receptor level, delaying progression and improving survival.

First attempt at maximum androgen blockade was by Huggins and Scott (1945) who performed bilateral adrenalectomies in four patients with metastatic prostate cancer. They all died from adrenal insufficiency.

In the early 1980s, Labrie reported increased survival time following total androgen blockade using Leuprolide and Flutamide. However, the trials lacked a control group and therefore the NCI carried out a randomized prospective study of Leuprolide and placebo versus Leuprolide and Flutamide in patients with metastatic prostate cancer. Crawford *et al.* studied 603 patients and found a significant difference in favour of combination therapy in terms of progression free survival and overall survival. The patients who received combination therapy had an improved survival of 7 months at 42 months follow-up. Although this study did not achieve the survival figures quoted by Labrie, the difference between the two groups was nevertheless significant. In addition, part of the enhanced survival reported by Crawford may be due to the ability of antiandrogens to neutralize the testosterone flare in the first 2 weeks following LHRH agonists.

An EORTC study (30853) compared orchidectomy with Goserelin and Flutamide in 327 patients with metastatic prostate cancer. Maximum androgen blockade resulted in significantly longer time to progression and significantly improved survival.

More recently, a meta-analysis of 5710 patients has failed to reveal a survival advantage from maximum androgen blockade and NCI intergroup study 0105 (comparing bilateral orchiectomy plus Flutamide to bilateral orchiectomy plus placebo) in 1387 patients found no survival advantage between the groups.

Antiandrogens are not without side effects and the clinician must balance the benefit in terms of survival from maximum androgen blockade with quality of life issues. The question remains as to the cost effectiveness of this expensive form of treatment in an ageing population.

Early versus late hormonal manipulation

Traditionally hormonal therapy for the treatment of metastatic prostate cancer has been delayed until the patient develops symptoms. This was based on the VACURG 1 study which failed to show a survival benefit in patients treated by orchidectomy or diethyl stilboestrol (DES) (5 mg/day) at time of diagnosis, compared to a placebo group. This study was flawed, not least by the fact that increased mortality due to the cardiovascular side effects of DES decreased survival in the early hormone manipulation group.

In the VACURG 2 study, a lower dose of DES (1mg/day) was used and patients receiving early hormonal manipulation did experience improved overall survival.

Data from the MRC trial of immediate versus deferred hormone manipulation in patients with locally advanced or metastatic prostate cancer have demonstrated a significant disease specific survival advantage in favour of those patients treated by early hormone manipulation. Nine hundred and thirty-eight patients with locally advanced or asymptomatic metastatic prostate cancer were randomized to either immediate treatment (BSO or LHRH analogue) or the same treatment deferred until an indication occurred. Ten year follow-up data on 934 patients are available. Progression to metastatic disease occurred more rapidly in deferred treatment group. Incidence of TURP, pathological fracture, cord compression, ureteric obstruction and extraskeletal metastasis was twice as high in the patients treated by deferred hormone manipulation. Results consistently favour immediate treatment.

Further reading

Crawford ED, Eisenberger MA, McLeod DG *et al.* (1989). A controlled trial of leuprolide with and without flutamide in prostatic carcinoma. *N Engl J Med*, **321**, 419–424.

Denis L, Smith P, De Moura JL *et al.* (1990). Orchidectomy versus Zoladex plus flutamide in patients with metastatic prostate cancer. The EORTC GU group. *Eur Urol*, **18**, 33–40.

Mayer FJ, Crawford MD (1993). Optimal therapy for metastatic prostate cancer. In: *Recent Advances in Urology/Andrology*, Vol. 6. (eds WF Hendry, RS Kirby) pp. 159–175. Churchill Livingstone, Edinburgh.

Prostate Cancer Trialists 'Collaborative Group' (1995). Maximum androgen blockade in advanced prostate cancer: an overview of 22 randomised trials with 3283 deaths in 5710 patients. *Lancet*, **346**, 265–269.

The Medical Research Council Prostate Cancer Working Party Investigators Group (1997). Immediate versus deferred treatment for advanced prostate cancer: initial results of the Medical Research Council Trial. *Br J Urol*, **79**, 235–246.

Bacillus Calmette–Guerin in the Treatment of Superficial Bladder Cancer

Introduction

- Bacillus Calmette–Guerin (BCG) was developed from a virulent strain of *Mycobacterium bovis* in 1908.
- It is a live attenuated organism.

- There are many commercially available strains which appear to have similar clinical activity, with the exception of Evans which is no longer in production, e.g. Connaught, Tice, Evans (Glaxo), Pasteur, RIV (Dutch).
- The correct dose is unclear; Lamm recommends 81 mg (dry weight Connaught). Solsona, however, has reported similar efficacy, with reduced toxicity, at a dose of 27 mg.

Mechanism of action
- BCG strains differ in their methods of production and preservation.
- The precise mechanism of action is unclear, but would appear to be mediated by a lymphocytic infiltrate and is T-cell dependent.
- The antitumour activity of BCG is most likely via enhanced immunological recognition of tumour in a manner similar to autoimmune disease.
- BCG organisms can persist in the urinary tract for up to 16.5 months after the completion of intravesical therapy.

Indications
- Carcinoma *in situ* (CIS) of the bladder.
- T1G3 transitional cell carcinoma of the bladder.
- Multiple recurrent Ta/T1 tumours not responding to Epirubicin or Mitomycin C.

CIS
- The role of BCG in CIS of the bladder is undisputed.
- If treated by resection alone CIS of the bladder progresses to muscle invasion in 60% of cases and one-third of patients are dead in 5 years.
- A meta-analysis of 18 published series reported an overall response rate for CIS of the bladder of 70% following six treatments over 6 weeks, increasing to 82% if an additional three instillations were given at 3 months.
- If no response is obtained after a single course of BCG it is reasonable to try a second course and a further 10% will respond, but a second failure is an indication for cystoprostatourethrectomy.

Maintenance therapy
- The SWOG study (8507) has shown that by the use of maintenance therapy (3 weekly instillations at 3 months, 6 months and every subsequent 6 months for 3 years) tumour free status can be maintained in 64–75% of cases for 5 years.

- When treated by a single course of BCG the relapse rate at 2 years is approximately 50%.
- Twenty-six per cent of patients on maintenance therapy had significant morbidity.

TIG3 tumours
- The risk of progression in T1 tumours can be as high as 50%, dependent on grade.
- T1G3 tumours warrant additional treatment to local resection in view of the risk of progression.
- In a meta-analysis of 309 patients, the overall risk of progression in T1 tumours was reduced from 35% to 13% following a single course of BCG.
- Some patients may find the risk of progression unacceptable and opt for immediate cystectomy.

Complications
- Following BCG therapy sloughing and denudation of the bladder mucosa is common.
- Intense inflammatory changes occur with infiltration of lamina propria by lymphocytes, plasma cells and polymorphonuclear cells.
- A transient sterile cystitis is common and granulomata may be reported on biopsy.
- Systemic infection has been reported in cases where recent resections have been performed prior to treatment and this has resulted in fatalities.
- Pulmonary infections along with localized infections of bladder, prostate and seminal vesicles have been reported many months after treatment.
- Cases of 'BCGosis' warrant antituberculous therapy.

Further reading
Bowyer L, Hall RR, Reading J, Marsh MM (1995). The persistence of bacille Calmette–Guerin in the bladder after intravesical treatment for bladder cancer. *Br J Urol*, **75**, 188–192.

Cookson MS, Sarosdy MF (1992). Management of stage 1 superficial bladder cancer with intraveiscal BCG therapy. *J Urol*, **148**, 797–801.

Lamm DL (1992). Carcinoma *in situ*. *Urol Clin North Am*, **19**, 499–508.

Kaisary AV (1991). BCG treatment for superficial bladder tumours. In: *Recent Advances in Urology/Andrology*, 5. pp. 119–133. Churchill Livingstone, Edinburgh.

Lamm DL (1992). Complications of BCG immunotherapy. *Urol Clin North Am*, **19**, 565–572.

Lamm DL, Blumenstein B, Sarosdy M, Grossman B, Crawford D (1997). Significant long term patient benefit with BCG maintenance therapy: a SWOG study. *J Urol* (Abs. 831), **157(4)**, 213.

Management of T1G3 Transitional Cell Carcinoma of the Bladder

Introduction
- pT1G3 tumours are, by definition, poorly differentiated and invade lamina propria. There is considerable intrapathologist variation in reporting. Specialist uropathologists disagree in up to 20% of cases.
- T1G3 tumours make up 12% of Ta/T1 tumours.
- Endoscopic treatment alone is inadequate. Treatment by resection alone results in a 5 year local recurrence rate of 60%.
- More worrying is the progression rate to invasion/metastasis which is approximately 40% (29–63%) and with concurrent CIS this risk has been reported as high as 80%.
- Cure rate: intravesical BCG approximately 50%; radical cystectomy approximately 90%.

Options for treatment
- Treatment options lie between immunotherapy, in the form of intravesical BCG therapy, and radical cystectomy.
- Intravesical chemotherapy is associated with a progression rate of 40%.
- Results from radiotherapy have been disappointing, particularly in the presence of associated CIS.
- Complete response rates following a single course of BCG have been reported to be between 59% and 82%. However, approximately 30% of these tumours will later progress, leaving about 50% 'cured'. Patients treated with a 6 week course of BCG who have persistent disease at 3 months are at high risk of disease progression (80%). Early cystectomy should be advised in these patients, provided they are fit for surgery. A second 6 week course of BCG may be offered in patients not fit for cystectomy and this may further increase response rates.
- If progression to muscle invasive disease does occur, the opportunity for cure may be lost. In a recent series of 23 patients with T1G3 tumours treated by intravesical BCG over a 10 year period, 74% had

local recurrence and 35% tumour progression. A further 22% of cases died from metastases despite salvage therapy. It is therefore important that both the urologist and the patient are aware of the potential risks of a bladder conserving approach.

- In the future it may be possible for the urologist to stratify patients according to risk of progression by the use of molecular markers such as p53, epidermal growth factor receptor or E-cadherin. For the time being, grade represents the most useful predictor of progression.

Further reading
Herr HW (1991). Progression of stage T1 bladder tumours after intravesical BCG. *J Urol*, **145**, 40–44.

Jakse G, Loidl W, Seeber G, Hofstadler H (1987). Stage 1 Grade 3 transitional cell carcinoma of the bladder. An unfavourable tumour. *J Urol*, **137**, 39–43.

Birch BR, Harlands SJ (1989). The pT1G3 bladder tumour. *Br J Urol*, **64**, 109–116.

Zhang GK, Uke ET, Sharer WC, Borkon WD, Bernstein SM (1996). Reassessment of conservative management for stage T1N0M0 transitional cell carcinoma of the bladder. *J Urol*, **155**, 1907–1909.

Radiotherapy in the Treatment of Bladder Cancer

Introduction
- Transitional cell carcinomas are radiosensitive, squamous cell carcinoma and adenocarcinoma respond less well (there are conflicting data as to the impact of squamous differentiation on the response to radiotherapy).
- Potentially cures one-third of patients with bladder conserved.
- Significant morbidity.
- Approximately 50% of tumours will recur locally at 5 years.

Traditionally radical radiotherapy was the preferred treatment for muscle invasive transitional cell carcinoma in the UK. However, with the development of reconstructive surgical techniques and increasing awareness of the morbidity and local recurrence rates associated with radiotherapy, cystectomy has become the first line treatment for muscle invasive bladder cancer. Although the bladder is preserved following radiotherapy, up to 70% of patients suffer from dysuria, frequency and diarrhoea. Approximately 10% will go on to develop chronic radiation cystitis.

External beam radiotherapy

- Radical external beam radiotherapy involves a dose of ≥60 Gy, usually given as a course of treatment over a 6 week period.
- This is followed by reassessment by cystoscopy and EUA, usually 3 months following treatment.
- Patients with stage T2 and T3 tumours may be treated provided there is no evidence of metastasis to local lymph nodes.
- Patients with T4a disease are best treated by radical surgery.
- Nodal disease is not sensitive to radiotherapy.
- Patients with more advanced disease (T4b) may be offered palliative radiotherapy at a reduced dose of 30–35 Gy.
- Approximately one-third of patients with muscle invasive disease confined to the bladder can be cured by radiotherapy alone. A further third will require salvage cystectomy for local recurrence and in the remaining third of patients disease will progress rapidly despite treatment.
- Five year survival rates for patients with T2–T3 bladder cancer range from 24–46% depending on stage (Gospodarowicz, 1989).
- Local recurrence rate following radiotherapy have been quoted as 50–70% compared to 10–20% following radical cystectomy. However, it is important to remember that most patients will die from distant metastases rather than local recurrence.
- Shipley has reviewed several large retrospective series and found that outcome was not only related to stage and grade but also to the degree to which the primary tumour was debulked by thorough TUR prior to radiotherapy.
- Patients with CIS or squamous differentiation may respond less well to radiotherapy.

Radiotherapy prior to cystectomy

During the late 1970s several centres explored the possibility of radiotherapy prior to cystectomy as a form of adjuvant treatment. In randomized studies no difference was demonstrated in terms of a survival benefit from preoperative treatment at 20–45 Gy. This treatment approach causes a delay in cystectomy and increases the morbidity of surgery.

Chemotherapy with radical radiotherapy

- It has been suggested that a combination of Cisplatin based chemotherapy and radiotherapy increases survival and local control.
- The first published randomized study comparing a combination of

radiotherapy and Cisplatin chemotherapy was the Canadian Bladder 3 study. No survival benefit was demonstrated, although local control was improved.

- The MRC/EORTC intercontinental study evaluating 3 cycles of neoadjuvant CMV in combination with radiotherapy/cystectomy again showed no survival advantage.

Further reading

Blandy JP, England HR, Evans SJ *et al.* (1980). T3 bladder cancer, the case for salvage cystectomy. *Br J Urol*, **52**, 506–510.

Bloom HJG, Hendry WF, Wallace DM, Skeet RG (1982). Treatment of T3 bladder cancer. Controlled trial of preoperative radiotherapy and radical cystectomy versus radical radiotherapy. *Br J Urol*, **54**, 136–151.

Gospodarowicz MK, Hawkins NV, Rawlings GA *et al.* (1989). Radical radiotherapy for muscle invasive transitional cell carcinoma of the bladder: failure analysis. *J Urol*, **142**, 1448–1454.

Jenkins BJ, Caulfied MJ, Fowler CG *et al.* (1988). Reappraisal of the role of radical radiotherapy and salvage cystectomy in the treatment of T2/T3 bladder cancer. *Br J Urol*, **62**, 343–346.

Shipley WU (1984). Full dose irradiation for invasive bladder carcinoma: prognostic factors and techniques. *Urology*, **33** (Suppl.), 95.

Fossa SD, Roberts T, Olsen DG (1997). Radiotherapy in the management of bladder cancer. In: *European Urology Update Series*, Vol. 6(4), pp. 80–85.

Chemotherapy for Transitional Cell Carcinoma of the Bladder

Introduction

- The prognosis for patients with invasive bladder cancer has not improved significantly over the past 30 years, most patients dying from metastatic disease.

- Patients with distant metastatic disease have a median survival of 6–9 months and those with regionally involved nodes have a median survival of 18 months.

- In order to improve survival in these patients it is necessary to develop successful systemic treatments.

- Transitional cell carcinoma of the bladder is unquestionably chemosensitive and response rates as high as 65% have been reported with complete response rates of 25%.

- Unfortunately this response is often short lived and relapse common.

Single agent chemotherapy
- The most active chemotherapeutic agents are Cisplatin, Methotrexate, Adriamycin and Vinblastine.
- Single agent chemotherapy has been used since the early 1960s when Methotrexate was reported to achieve response rates of up to 30%.
- Cisplatin is the most active single agent and response rates as high as 40% have been reported.
- Adriamycin has significant activity (20% response rates) and its less cardiotoxic derivative Epirubicin has similar activity.
- Vinblastine is the least active single agent achieving response rates of 15%.

Combination chemotherapy
- Combination chemotherapy regimens evolved during the 1980s.
- MVAC was developed by the Memorial Sloan Kettering group, CMV by Stanford University and the North Carolina Oncology group.
- The CISCA regimen was popularized by the MD Anderson group, but response rates were not as high as MVAC and CMV.
- The initial results from these treatment regimens were very optimistic (response rate MVAC 70%, CMV 56%) but with longer follow-up relapse was common.
- Durability of response appears to be longer for MVAC (median 38 months) than CMV (median 14 months). In retrospect, some of the patients labelled clinical complete responders may not have been staged correctly as they did not have resection biopsies performed, which is now mandatory to establish true complete response.

Metastatic disease
- Combination therapy may be offered to patients with metastatic disease with adequate renal function.
- Durable remissions may be achieved in up to 20% of cases and a small but significant survival advantage has been reported in randomized studies.
- Patients with visceral metastases are less likely to respond than those with purely nodal metastases.
- MVAC is more toxic than CMV but response rates are higher.

Adjuvant therapy
- Patients with locally advanced bladder cancer, positive nodes or with evidence of vascular/lymphatic invasion may be offered adjuvant therapy in addition to radical surgery or radiotherapy.

- Skinner has reported increased survival in patients receiving mainly adjuvant Cisplatin, Doxorubicin and Cyclophosphamide following radical cystectomy in a non-randomized study. The only randomized study from Germany closed too early for satisfactory statistical analysis.

Neoadjuvant therapy
- This term refers to primary chemotherapy as a first line means of treatment.
- In the most successful cases, complete resolution of tumour may occur but more often the result is down staging of disease prior to cystectomy.
- MVAC can lead to response rates of 70% and as many as 33% of cases have no tumour demonstrated at cystectomy.
- A meta-analysis of neoadjuvant Cisplatin based chemotherapy has shown no survival benefit.
- Data from the recent MRC/EORTC intercontinental randomized study (975 patients) also shows no survival benefit from 3 cycles of CMV.

New agents
- Improvements in therapy of advanced transitional cell carcinoma are unlikely to come from existing regimens.
- Data from accelerated dosing regimens in combination with human granulocyte stimulating factor have been disappointing.
- New agents are under evaluation such as Piritrexim, Paclitaxel, Gallium nitrate, Ifosfamide and Gemcitabine.

Further reading
Arap W, Scher HI (1992). Cytotoxic chemotherapy for locally advanced and metastatic bladder cancer. In: *Urological Oncology* (eds J Waxman, G Williams), pp. 185–199. Edward Arnold, London.

Ghersi D, Stewart LA, Parmar MKB *et al.* (1995). Advanced bladder cancer overview collaboration. Does neoadjuvant cisplatin based chemotherapy improve the survival of patients with locally advanced bladder cancer: a meta-analysis of individual data from randomised clinical trials. *Br J Urol*, **75**, 206–213.

Roth BJ, Bajorin DF (1995). Advanced bladder cancer: the need to identify new agents in the post MVAC world. *J Urol*, **153**, 894–900.

Sternberg CN, Yagoda A, Scher HI (1988). MVAC for advanced transitional cell carcinoma of the urothelium. *J Urol*, **139**, 461–469.

Skinner DG, Daniels JR, Russel CA *et al.* (1991). The role of adjuvant chemotherapy following cystectomy for invasive bladder cancer: a prospective comparative trial. *J Urol*, **145**, 459–467.

Andrology

Surgery for Impotence

Introduction

The majority of older men presenting with impotence will have both organic (mainly vascular) and psychological factors. Most cases (60–80%) can be successfully managed using non-operative methods including psychosexual therapy, vacuum/constriction devices and injection pharmacotherapy. Surgical options are prosthesis insertion or corrective vascular surgery to restrict outflow or increase inflow.

Prosthetic implants

- Malleable: semi-rigid silicone rods.
- Three piece inflatable: cylinders, pump, reservoir.
- One piece inflatable: cylinders only.

This is a treatment option for predominant organic impotence in well motivated couples who have been extensively counselled and any psychological component treated; most will have tried and failed with other forms of therapy. Inflatable devices are not suitable if severe corporal fibrosis is present. Most couples need a 6–12 month adjustment period following implantation.

Counselling

- Length and girth less than natural erection.
- Altered sensation and ejaculatory failure (5–10%).
- Risk of infection.
- Difficulties with concealment.
- Use of silicone.

Malleable rods

- Low cost.
- Simple to insert through distal corporotomies with circumcision.
- Infection rate 0.6–9% (increased risk in diabetics, men with spinal cord injury, second implantations).
- Seventy-five per cent have evidence of silicone particles in surrounding lymphatics.
- Mechanical failure 0%.
- Patient satisfaction 70–75%.

- Partner satisfaction 40–50%.
- Eighty per cent use the device for sexual intercourse.

Three piece devices
- High cost.
- Good detumescence.
- Implanted via infrapubic or penoscrotal approach.
- Mechanical failure 2–30% (average 5%).
- Infection 0.8–9%.
- Patient satisfaction 70–90%.
- Partner satisfaction 70%.
- >90% use device.

One piece devices
- High mechanical failure rate 18–26%.
- Patient satisfaction 60%.

Venous surgery
- Dorsal vein ligation described by Lydston in 1908.
- Ligation of dorsal vein and veins arising from corpora cavernosa.
- Ligation of dorsal vein, corporal veins and plication of crura (Lowsley's operation reported by Millin in 1936).

These operations were developed at a time when penile erection was thought to occur by complete penile venous occlusion. Early publications suggested a 50–60% response rate in unselected men. The concept of 'venous leak' diagnosed by cavernosometry and cavernosography rekindled interest in this type of surgery in the 1980s.

Results
- Early response rates: at 1 year up to 50% better or cured.
- Long-term results: at 2–5 years 20% have benefit.

Haemodynamic changes necessary for erection are now thought to be dependent upon adequate inflow and cavernosal smooth muscle relaxation. Partial passive occlusion of emissary veins traversing the tunica albuginea may occur. The finding of 'venous leakage' is probably due to cavernosal smooth muscle failure. Venous ligation surgery has therefore largely been discarded as an option for the treatment of impotence.

Arterial surgery
- Inferior epigastric to corpus cavernosum (Michal I 1973).
- Inferior epigastric to dorsal artery (Michal II 1980).
- Inferior epigastric to deep dorsal vein (Virag 1980).

- Inferior epigastric to dorsal artery and deep dorsal vein (Hauri 1984).

The demonstration of distal pudendal and common penile arterial stenoses in impotent men by arteriography and colour duplex ultrasonography encouraged the development of microsurgical corporal revascularization in the hope of increasing inflow to the corpora during erection.

Results
- Patency rates 80%.
- Early response rates: at 1 year 50–60% better or cured.
- Long-term results: at 2–5 years 30–40% better or cured.
- Young men with arterial damage post-pelvic fractures: 80% success.

Older men who fail to respond to intracavernosal drugs are likely to have cavernosal smooth muscle failure limiting the usefulness of arterial surgery. Most centres would only offer such surgery to men < 60 years old with localized bilateral arterial occlusion, no diabetes and no other evidence of peripheral or coronary atherosclerotic disease.

Further reading

Freedman AL, Costa Neto F, Mehringer CM, Rajfer J (1993). Long-term results of penile vein ligation for impotence from venous leakage. *J Urol*, **149**, 1301–1303.

Cookson MS, Phillips DL, Huff ME, Fitch WP (1993). Analysis of microsurgical revascularization results by aetiology of impotence. *J Urol*, **149**, 1308–1312.

Lewis RW (1995). Long-term results of penile prosthetic implants. *Urol Clin North Am*, **22**, 847–856.

Kabalin JN, Kuo JC (1997) Long term followup and patient satisfaction with the Dynaflex self-contained inflatable penile prosthesis. *J Urol*, **158**, 456–459.

Semen Analysis

Introduction
Traditional semen parameters used in the investigation of infertile couples include sperm density, morphology and motility. Subnormal values roughly correlate with pregnancy rates but more sophisticated measurements are necessary to classify sperm dysfunction. In an attempt to improve quality control and standardize methodology, guidelines for semen collection, analysis and interpretation have been formulated by the World Health Organization (WHO). Sperm density and quality show a gradual decline over the last 50 years in most populations but the cause is uncertain.

Ejaculate
- Sample collection
  set period of abstinence;
  complete ejaculate collected in a sterile non-toxic container;
  rapid transfer to the laboratory;
  repeated samples over a 3 month period if abnormal.
- Volume > 2 ml.
- Coagulation followed by reliquefaction.
- Low volume, lack of coagulation and low pH (with low fructose) indicates lack of seminal vesicular fluid (associated with ejaculatory duct obstruction).

Sperm density
- Ejaculate diluted with phenol to stop motility.
- Counted with a graticule and expressed as sperm/ml and total sperm.
- Normal >20 million/ml; <10 million/ml almost certain subfertility.
- Fifty thousand are needed for *in vitro* fertilization (IVF), single sperm for direct oocyte injection.

Sperm motility
- Normal > 50% showing forward movement.
- Correlation with fertilization rates is poor.

Sperm morphology
- Stage of development.
- Morphological abnormalities of the head, mid-piece and tail.
- Acrosome status.
- Normal > 50% intact mature sperm.
- Best predictor of sperm function and overall fertility.

Immunology
- Inflammatory cells
  significance is uncertain;
  normal < 1 million/ml.
- Antisperm autoantibodies
  present in serum, seminal plasma or bound to sperm;
  IgG or IgA;
  3–15% of infertile men;
  detected by mixed agglutination reaction or microbead;
  significant levels if positive result at dilution > 1/64.

Sperm function
- For couples considering assisted conception.
- Cervical mucus penetration tested by exposing sperm to partner and donor mucus. Normal result suggested by > 16–20 motile sperm per high power field in alkaline mucus.
- Capacitation (formation of acrosome) tested by D-manose ligand binding.
- Acrosome reaction tested by comparing binding and reaction of partner and donor sperm with hemizona preparations from donor oocyte. Normally should have spontaneous acrosomal loss and high induced acrosomal response.
- Assay of successful sperm penetration of hamster ova.

Further reading
Nieschlag E (1993). Care for the infertile male. *Clin Endocrinol*, **38**, 123–133.
Bar-Chama N, Lamb DJ (1994). Evaluation of sperm function. What is available in the modern andrology laboratory. *Urol Clin North Am*, **21**, 433–446.

Treatment of Oligospermia

Introduction
Oligospermia is defined as sperm density persistently < 20 million/ml. It is usually associated with poor motility (oligoaesthenospermia) and structural defects (oligoteratospermia). Because sperm are present, female factors must be investigated and treated whilst the man is being assessed. In addition it should be established that the couple's sexual activity and understanding of the reproductive cycle is sufficient for conception.

Aetiology
- Testicular damage
  cryptorchidism
  torsion
  varicocoele
  infection.
- Toxins
  alcohol, tobacco, marijuana
  drugs, including anabolic steroids, Sulphasalazine and Cimetidine
  chemotherapy and radiotherapy.

- Hyperthermia
  underwear
  pyrexial illness.
- Occupational
  pesticides
  heavy metals.
- Idiopathic
  approximately 30% of cases associated with mild elevation of follicle stimulating hormone (FSH).

Varicocoele ablation

- Associated with small ipsilateral testis and progressively impaired semen parameters.
- Ablation improves semen parameters.
- Thirty to 40% pregnancy rates in early uncontrolled studies.
- Randomized trials have shown no benefit if female factors adequately treated.
- Indication for ablation: men with clinically apparent varicocoele confirmed on ultrasound with smaller ipsilateral testis and subnormal semen parameters, and normal or treated partner.
- Controlled studies show similar pregnancy rates following embolization or high/inguinal/laparoscopic ligation. Embolization has lesser incidence of testicular arterial damage and hydrocoele.

Hormonal therapy

- Trials lack placebo arms to control for 20–40% spontaneous pregnancy rate.
- Three to 6 months of treatment necessary to cover at least one sperm maturation/delivery cycle.
- Gonadotrophin therapy ineffective.
- Anti-oestrogens or testolactone (aromatase inhibitor), given to decrease negative effect of oestrogens on luteinizing hormone (LH) secretion, have been used but results are inconclusive.

Steroids

- Used in men with high serum or seminal antisperm antibody titre.
- Controversial.
- Moderate doses (10–20 mg Prednisolone) given for 7–10 days around ovulation for 9 months; decreased side effects and resulted in improved pregnancy rates.
- Shorter treatment schedules show no effect.

Assisted conception
- Inferior results in male factor infertility.
- Sperm preparation
  seminal plasma removed;
  sperm washed and motile sperm selected;
  induction of capacitation.
- Intrauterine insemination
  during ovulation;
  no definite benefit over natural intercourse;
  can be combined with stimulated ovulation;
  indicated if sperm penetration assay normal.
- *In vitro* fertilization
  retrieval of mature oocytes;
  in vitro insemination with processed sperm;
  reimplantation of embryos;
  lower fertilization rates in male factor infertility (23% versus 71%);
  improved by additional sperm processing to 50%;
  abnormal morphology associated with high rate of miscarriage.
- Direct injection of sperm
  partial zonal dissection;
  subzonal insertion of sperm (SZI);
  intracytoplasmic sperm injection (ICSI);
  pregnancy rates of up to 35%.

Further reading

Hendry WF, Hughes L, Scammell G, Prior JP, Hargreave TB (1990). Comparison of prednisolone and placebo in subfertile men with antibodies to spermatozoa. *Lancet*, **335**, 85–88.

Bals-Pratch M, Doren M, Karbowski B, Schneider HPG, Nieschlag E (1992). Cyclic corticosteroid immunosuppression is unsuccessful in the treatment of sperm antibody-related male infertility: a controlled study. *Hum Reprod*, 7, 99–104.

Ross LS, Ruppman N (1993). Varicocele vein ligation in 565 patients under local anaesthesia: a long-term review of technique, results and complications in light of proposed management by laparoscopy. *J Urol*, **149**, 1361–1363.

Sigman M (1994). Assisted reproduction techniques and male infertility. *Urol Clin North Am*, **21**, 505–515.

Schlesinger MH, Wilets IF, Nagler HM (1994). Treatment outcome after varicocelectomy. *Urol Clin North Am*, **21**, 517–529.

Intersex

Introduction
Intersex states are characterized by the presence of ambiguous genitalia following disordered fetal sexual differentiation. Gender of an individual is a composite of chromosomal, gonadal and phenotypic sex.

Physiology
- Default sex is female.
- Modified by presence of testis determining factor gene (TDF, a DNA binding protein) on short arm of Y chromosome (Yp).
- Interaction between X, Y and autosomal genes.
- TDF stimulates formation of seminiferous tubules, Sertoli cells and Leydig cells.
- Testosterone (T) released by Leydig cells at 8 weeks in response to placental hCG.
- Sertoli cells secrete Mullerian inhibiting factor (MIF).
- Without TDF oogonia form and Mullerian system persists (20 weeks).
- T and MIF act by passive diffusion on ipsilateral target tissues.
- Male external genitalia require peripheral conversion of T to dihydrotestosterone (DHT).
- Penile shaft development from urethral fold is complex and prone to abnormality.
- T surge in neonate ensures testicular descent and possibly male behavioural patterns.
- Puberty results from hypothalamic/pituitary activation with nocturnal gonadotrophin secretion.

Female pseudohermaphroditism
- Virilization of the external genitalia of a female (46XX) fetus.
- Normal ovaries and hence no palpable gonads.
- Variable phenotype.
- Congenital adrenal hyperplasia (CAH)
  21-hydroxylase type
  autosomal recessive
  salt loss in 50%
  excess adrenal androgens.
- Maternal androgens.

Male pseudohermaphroditism
- Incomplete virilization of a male (46XY) fetus.

- Normal testes present (may be undescended).
- Wolffian structures are underdeveloped or absent.
- Further virilization at puberty also impaired.
- Mullerian structures absent (normal MIF).
- Variable phenotype: ranges from female genitalia to severe hypospadias alone.
- Impaired Leydig cell activity
  inborn errors of T biosynthesis
  hypoplastic Leydig cells.
- 5α-reductase deficiency: normal internal genitalia.
- Androgen receptor defects
  defective expression of androgen receptor gene on Xq
     due to point mutations of steroid binding domain;
  variable phenotype;
  complete testicular feminization presents as primary
     amenorrhoea. Higher risk of testicular cancer;
  incomplete feminization and Reifenstein's syndrome
     have perineal hypospadias;
  infertile male syndrome with normal phenotype.

Gonadal dysgenesis
- Impaired gonadal differentiation.
- Mixed gonadal dysgenesis
  cryptorchid testis with contralateral streak gonad;
  46XY or 45XO/46XY mosaic karyotype;
  phenotype shows partial virilization on testis side and
     contralateral Mullerian structures;
  high risk of testicular malignancy in female phenotype.
- True hermaphrodites
  rare; have both spermatogonia and oogonia;
  46XX or mosaic;
  single palpable gonad usually an ovotestis.

Clinical features
- Ambiguous genitalia: hypospadias, cryptorchidism, clitoral hypertrophy.
- Palpable scrotal gonads
  two indicates male pseudohermaphroditism; serum T
     will reveal cause;
  one with asymmetry suggests gonadal dysgenesis;
  none indicates female pseudohermaphroditism.
- Other developmental anomalies.

- Karyotyping: T-lymphocytes from peripheral blood.
- Pelvic ultrasound: Mullerian structures and gonads.
- Laparoscopy: Mullerian structures and gonads/vas.
- Hormonal and enzyme assays.
- hCG stimulation test: measurement of T/DHT to assess testicular function.
- Androgen binding: assayed using cultured fibroblasts.
- Complete assessment reveals chromosomal, gonadal and phenotypic sex with likely aetiology of disorder.

Treatment
- Choice of gender
  should await the outcome of investigation;
  depends upon likely fertility, phenotypic appearance and feasibility of reassignment.
- Hormonal
  T/DHT or LH therapy if androgen deficient;
  steroids for salt loss.
- Surgery
  orchidopexy or remove gonads;
  excision of Mullerian structures and vagina, or clitoral reduction and vaginoplasty;
  repair hypospadias.

Further reading
Pagon RA (1987). Diagnostic approach to the new-born with ambiguous genitalia. *Pediatr Clin North Am*, **34**, 1019–1031.
Savage MO (1989). Clinical aspects of intersex. In: *Clinical Paediatric Endocrinology* (ed. CGD Brook), pp. 38–54. Blackwell, Oxford.
Jaffe T, Oates RD (1994). Genetic abnormalities and reproductive failure. *Urol Clin North Am*, **21**, 389–408.

Treatment of Priapism

Introduction
Priapism is a long-recognized condition characterized by persistent erection in the absence of sexual stimulation. Pain and tenderness usually occur and the condition is not relieved by orgasm. An excellent descriptive case report given by a London surgeon, JW Tripe (1845) is well worth reading.

Classification
- High flow
  uncommon;
  persistent arteriolar dilatation or arterio-venous fistula.
- Low flow
  most frequent;
  persistent cavernosal relaxation.
- Primary
  no identifiable cause in 50% of cases.
- Secondary
  drugs, including intracavernosal therapy and neuroleptics;
  sickle cell disease in up to 20% of cases;
  haematological malignancies;
  neurogenic in men with spinal cord injury.

Clinical features
- Usually occurs during sleep (80%) or following sexual activity (17%).
- Involves cavernous bodies not corpus spongiosum or glans.
- Low flow
  rigid cool penis;
  venous blood gas picture on aspiration;
  high risk of fibrosis (irreversible >24 hours).
- High flow
  history of recent or previous trauma;
  rigid pulsatile penis;
  arterial blood gas picture on aspiration;
  low risk of fibrosis.
- Intracavernosal drugs
  younger men with better baseline erectile function;
  neurological impotence;
  papaverine > prostaglandin E_1 or phentolamine.

Investigation
- history
- haematological investigation
- cavernosal blood gas analysis
- colour duplex ultrasound and arteriography in high flow cases.

Treatment
- All cases
  analgesia and anxiolytics;

aspiration of corpora via 19 swg butterfly needle;
irrigation with α-agonist, e.g. 10 mg Phenylephrine in 500 ml saline.
* High flow
pudendal arteriography with embolization;
open ligation of abnormal vessels;
no treatment may give better long-term outcome.
* Low flow
cavernosospongiosal shunt;
Winter (1976): fenestrate tunica albuginea with biopsy needle via glans;
Ebbehoj (1975): incise tunica via glans;
Ercole (1981): excise window of tunica via glans;
Quackels (1964): proximal open cavernosospongiosal shunt if distal
fibrosis or glanular shunt fails;
saphenous shunt of no benefit.
* Sickle cell
exchange transfusion;
surgery gives higher risk of impotence.

Outcome
* Recurrence 10–60%, especially idiopathic and sickle cell.
* Fibrosis in low flow priapism; tissue changes begin at 12 hours,
fibroblast activity at 48 hours.
* Impotence 10–40%; increased following surgical intervention to 50%.
* Conservative management may be best option in haematological and
high flow states.
* Surgery required with prolonged idiopathic low flow priapism.

Further reading

Tripe JW (1845) Case of continued priapism *Lancet*, **2**, 8–9.

Winter CC (1978). Priapism cured by creation of fistulas between the glans penis
and corpora cavernosa. *J Urol*, **119**, 227–228.

Ercole CJJ, Pontes JE, Pierce JM (1981). Changing surgical concepts in the
treatment of priapism. *J Urol*, **125**, 210–211.

Pohl J, Pott B, Kleinhans G (1986). Priapism: a three phase concept of management
according to aetiology and prognosis. *Br J Urol*, **58**, 113–118.

Witt MA, Goldstein I, Saenz de Tejada I *et al.* (1990). Traumatic laceration of
intracavernosal arteries: the pathophysiology of non-ischaemic high flow arterial
priapism. *J Urol*, **143**, 129–132.

Surgical Treatment of Peyronie's Disease

Introduction
Peyronie's disease is characterized by the development of fibrotic plaque(s) in the tunica albuginea that envelop the corpora cavernosa. It most commonly affects the dorsal penile surface (80%) and causes curvature and axial distortion on erection.

Aetiology
- Uncertain.
- Sexual trauma.
- Fibrous dysplasia: associated with Dupuytren's contracture.
- Infection.
- Pathology: decreased elastic fibres, vasculitis, chronic inflammatory infiltrate.

Natural history
- Spontaneous resolution: 13–50% of cases over a 4 year period.
- Progression: 40% with increasing diffuse plaque formation.
- Stable disease.
- Impotence secondary to tunical, smooth muscle or arterial dysfunction.

Selection for surgery
- Required in 10–30% of cases.
- Observed for 18 month–2 year period to ensure stable deformity.
- Artificial erection test or home photograph to document deformity and rigidity.
- Penile straightening: significant curvature preventing enjoyment of intercourse with normal erectile rigidity.
- Plaque incision and graft: severe complex deformity and/or short penis.
- Prosthesis insertion: diffuse fibrosis, complete or distal flaccidity, penile shortening unacceptable to patient.

Nesbit operation
- Originally described for congenital curvature.
- Artificial erection induced with saline and tourniquet or PGE_1.
- Penis degloved.
- Ellipses of tunica opposite deformity excised (plication alone probably adequate).
- Defects closed transversely.

- Artificial erection repeated; any residual deformity corrected by plicating sutures.
- Penile shortening of 1–2cm and risk of 'waisting'.
- Patient satisfaction 70% if potent preoperatively (decreases with longer follow-up).
- Impotence 3–28%.
- Intracavernosal drugs can be used to augment erectile response.

Plaque excision/incision
- Excision or transverse 'H'-shaped incision of the plaque.
- Careful preservation of dorsal neurovascular bundles.
- Grafting with dermis, Gortex, dorsal vein, saphenous vein or pedicled preputial onlay.
- Glans hypothesia 10–50%.
- Patient satisfaction 60–70%.
- Impotence rate 30–100%.

Implants
- Straightening of penis with multiple plaque incisions or fractures.
- Grafting of defects if necessary.
- Malleable implant best if corporal fibrosis present.
- No penile shortening.
- High patient satisfaction.

Overview
The balance of evidence favours the Nesbit operation or simple plication for men with good erectile rigidity, although about 20% will have a decline in potency following surgery. Plaque incision and grafting causes less penile shortening but risks altered glanular sensation. A penile implant gives excellent patient satisfaction for those with erectile failure or severe deformity.

Further reading
Frank JD, Mor SB, Pryor JP (1981). The surgical correction of erectile deformities of the penis' of 100 men. *Br J Urol*, **53**, 645–647.

Gelbard MK, Dorey F, James K (1990). The natural history of Peyronie's disease. *J Urol*, **144**, 1376–1379.

O'Donnell PD (1992). Results of surgical management of Peyronie's disease. *J Urol*, **148**, 1184–1187.

Poulsen J, Kirkeby HJ (1995). Treatment of penile curvature: a retrospective study of 175 patients operated with either plication of the tunica albuginea or with the Nesbit procedure. *Br J Urol*, **75**, 370–374.

Index